Mountebanks and Medicasters

Mountebanks and Medicasters

A History of Italian Charlatans
from the Middle Ages
to the Present

PIERO GAMBACCINI

Translated by Bettie Gage Lippitt
Foreword by Giorgio Cosmacini

McFarland & Company, Inc., Publishers
Jefferson, North Carolina, and London

Originally published as *I Mercanti della Salute: le segrete virtù dell'-imbroglio in medicina* by Casa Editrice le Lettere, Florence (2002).

LIBRARY OF CONGRESS CATALOGUING-IN-PUBLICATION DATA

Gambaccini, Piero.
    Mountebanks and medicasters : a history of Italian charlatans
from the middle ages to the present / Piero Gambaccini ; translated
by Bettie Gage Lippitt ; foreword by Giorgio Cosmacini.
        p.   cm.
    Includes bibliographical references and index.

    ISBN 0-7864-1606-8 (softcover : 50# alkaline paper)

    1. Quacks and quackery — Italy — History.
    2. Medicine — Italy — History.   I. Title.
    R730.G24   2004
    615.8'56'0945 — dc22   2003021722

British Library cataloguing data are available

Cover art: *I ciarlatani in Piazzetta*, Gabriel Bella, oil on cloth, 57½" × 37",
1750 *(Querini Stampalia Foundation, Venice)*

Manufactured in the United States of America

McFarland & Company, Inc., Publishers
  Box 611, Jefferson, North Carolina 28640
    www.mcfarlandpub.com

To my father, who healed his patients
with a physician's science and a charlatan's art.

Acknowledgments

For the most part, the historical sources were found in the State Archives of Florence, Venice, Siena and Naples; the Biblioteca Nazionale Centrale in Florence; the Biblioteca Marciana in Venice; the Institute for the History of Medicine at the University of Rome; the collections of the Wellcome Institute for the History of Medicine in London; and the Rare Book Room of the New York Academy of Medicine.

My heartfelt thanks for their invaluable contribution in researching this book go to Dr. Giuseppe Parigino of the University of Florence; Dr. Franco Boschi of the University of Rome; Dr. Adriana Di Domenico of the Biblioteca Nazionale in Florence; and Alessandra Cavazzana in Venice. But I am especially indebted to Bettie, my wife and translator, for her constant help and essential suggestions and for having reined in, with Anglo-Saxon pragmatism, my runaway chatter.

Table of Contents

Foreword

In the vast archives of Simancas, which house the records of the Spanish Empire — that realm on which "the sun never set" — it is possible to make an intriguing discovery: Written in the margin of a memorandum by King Philip IV (1605–1665) is the apparently sibylline phrase: "Charlar es ablàr de ciencia." The regal comment seems to imply that when charlatans chatter they speak of wisdom, which supports the premise that, in centuries past, the term "charlatan" had a meaning that was anything but defamatory. Over the centuries, the charlatan had a role in healing that was not lacking in a certain dignity. In contrast to an official medicine that claimed to know and to be able to cure all, when actually it knew very little and was able to cure almost nothing, charlatans, in spite of all their boasting and eccentricities, answered in their own way an irrepressible and primary human need: the need to find a remedy, even if only consolatory, for disease, old age, and the fear of death. In this context, the charlatan was a product of mankind's existential anguish and of his anxiousness to live.

But he was not only this. The tooth drawer, capable of removing teeth and pain, the bonesetter who could adjust a dislocated shoulder with his hands, the dealer in remedies which were perhaps only made of beneficial suggestion, somehow answered the needs of a very large part of society which erudite medicine in fact precluded from any assistance. Unavoidably, amongst these merit-worthy charlatans thrived many self-styled healers who, taking advantage of the gullibility of the populace, exchanged malpractice for popular medicine.

The seventeenth century was not only a century of triumphant quackery, nor was it only a century of recurring plague and Baroque architecture. It was also the century of the "scientific revolution," of Galileo's new mechanics, of Harvey's cardiocirculatory physiology, of Malpighi's "inge-

1

nious and subtle anatomy," of Boyle's protochemistry. The period's ambiguity is reflected in ambiguous personages, as often accused of being charlatans as they were celebrated as innovators— men in good or bad faith, whose vicissitudes, often adventurous, were sometimes marked by clamorous defeat, and other times by an equally clamorous success.

When the Sun King asked Molière, who knew physicians well, what was the secret of the doctor who was curing him, the playwright answered, "Sire, we converse." Since the beginning of time, medical cures are also made not of useless chatter but of good words well said; since recent times cures are also made from clinically and epidemiologically verified experiments. Without these medical-anthropological and scientific-technical bases, medicine reverts to quackery. But the irrepressible need of the sick to search for remedies that will assuage their own fears and lighten the burdens of existence fuel the conviction in many that these remedies can be found beyond the limits of science and beyond the limits of their own bodies. In any period, those physicians who take advantage of these beliefs by practicing a medicine that is beyond the bounds of a science intended to serve mankind, and beyond the confines of medical ethics, are without any worth.

This book explores this world, during an arc of time that, centered on the seventeenth century, returns in part to the preceding centuries and is protracted into the centuries that followed. It is a fascinating book. Its fascination derives from the subject treated and the style of the author; it teaches while amusing, and in accordance with good historical method, it leads us to understand the problems of our present through the reconstruction of a controversial past. The result is excellent.

Giorgio Cosmacini
Fall 2003

Giorgio Cosmacini holds degrees both in medicine and philosophy. Like the author of this book, his specialization is radiology. He is currently Professor of the Department of the History of Medicine at the University of Milan. He is also head of the editorial board of the publishers Laterza (Rome and Bari) and Einaudi (Turin). He is the author of numerous books, including a three-volume History of Medicine and Health in Italy *(Laterza).*

Preface

In 1967, Dr. Christian Barnard performed his first heart transplant, one of the most revolutionary surgical feats in the history of medicine. About two years later, he was invited to an international medical congress in Florence. The president of the congress asked Barnard to examine a group of children afflicted with congenital cardiac disease, and as a radiologist with experience in this field, I was contacted to assist him. The lanky and boyish young doctor had by that time become a world celebrity, hounded by journalists, sought after by social hostesses, chased by movie actresses, and followed everywhere by crowds of people who hoped to touch or at least catch a glimpse of him. For two afternoons we were closeted in an office of a private clinic, while the police kept the curious at bay and Barnard visited his small patients. As each child was brought in, I handed the famous doctor a stack of X-rays regarding the case; during one of these exchanges, he dropped the whole pile on the floor. As we stooped to gather them up, I noticed that he seemed to have difficulty moving the fingers of his left hand. When he saw my puzzled gaze, he confessed in a low voice that he believed that he had rheumatoid arthritis, a disease that would soon have prevented him from practicing surgery. I asked him if he had tried all the therapies that were currently recommended, and he answered that he had, with very negligible results. Then he told me with a rueful smile that the only cure that had given him any relief at all was that of a healer, a pranotherapist.

I kept his secret until his premature death, but I often wondered how the most illustrious surgeon in the world had been attracted to, and had even obtained some benefit from, an unorthodox healer. I became convinced that even in our own time, in a century of transplants and huge medical advances, the hopes and fears and needs of the sick are not very different

3

from those of the masses of centuries past who stood in the squares, bare-foot and openmouthed, listening to the promises of medical charlatans.

Reminded of an encounter that had occurred many years before between my father, who was just beginning his first medical practice, and a shrewd charlatan, I became intrigued with this age-old popular counter-part to medicine, a cultural tradition that is often denied and neglected. In history books that recount medicine's slow and laborious progress, charlatanism is mentioned in a few hurried lines, dealt with like a sister of ill repute of whom to be ashamed. Medical literature gives only an accusatory description of quackery, considered a fearful impediment to knowledge, an unhealthy perversion of the human spirit. The medical charlatan's trade is presented as a deceitful act that takes place between a rogue without scruples and his victim, a person with a weak, simple, and credulous mind.

When I began my research for this book, I became fascinated with the history of quackery in Italy. I was surprised to discover that only a few vague and uncertain mentions of this ancient art existed before the fifteenth century, for the boundaries between quackery and orthodox med-icine were so faded and uncertain that one often trespassed into the field of the other. I therefore had to begin with the centuries in which Euro-pean universities began teaching medicine, a time in which it was decreed by law that only licensed physicians could practice. With their diplomas, physicians acquired a corporate right that gave them a monopoly on heal-ing, a right that was protected by the medical colleges, whose duty it was to defend licensed physicians from unorthodox healers. From the very beginning, an opposing dualism was created between the charlatan and the learned doctor, as if between vice and virtue, ignorance and knowledge. These unlicensed healers enraged medical doctors, who feared and hated their competition, not only for rational or moral reasons but for an ill-con-cealed desire to protect their own corporate interests.

My investigation took me seven years, and led me from the fifteenth century right up to our own times. I sifted through medical treatises and histories, hoping to discover between the lines the practices, always described as fraudulent, of medical charlatans. Records regarding quacks are often fragmentary and incomplete, subjected to the prejudices of the dominant medical establishment. While doctors were usually represented as heroes in the struggle against ignorance, charlatans were generally considered a pack of scoundrels for whom "shackles and chains would be fitting," at least in the opinion of Anton Francesco Bertini, a learned seventeenth-century professor of medicine.

The archives of most Italian cities contain not only government records and countless edicts enacted to hinder the charlatans' activities, but also stories of the endless encounters between the sly and the foolish in amusing chronicles of village and farm life and in the annals of noble courts. Spidery and faded calligraphies record the proceedings of trials and convictions, the petitions to those in power, the protests of doctors and pharmacists, the testimonials of gratitude on the part of beneficiaries and the remonstrances of those who had been deceived. These often dusty and forgotten documents describe the activities of ranks of Italian charlatans, some dashing and elegant, all endowed with a talent for irony and an unending ability to mock their fellows.

Italian medical charlatans, wandering quacks who traded in remedies, dogged official medicine throughout its slow and difficult progress. For centuries, they were the most numerous, the most sought after, and the most imitated quacks in all the countries of Europe. Absolute masters of the city and village squares, they attracted the crowds with their grandiloquent spiels from the height of a platform, enchanted the public with their witticisms, amused them, like consummate plebeian actors, with fantastic spectacles. These sly and easygoing enchanters contrived their ingenious tricks with imagination and presented their spectacles with a perverse taste for paradox.

While licensed physicians high-handedly prescribed cataclysmic enemas, drastic emetics, exhausting purges and merciless bloodlettings, the charlatans sold simple remedies that all could afford, accompanying them with words of hope and consoling promises. They were not only a throng of fraudulent quacks committed to swindling a gullible and ingenuous rabble; often, theirs was a form of opposition to a false, arrogant and presumptuous academic medicine. Sometimes, new and courageous ideas were hidden beneath their ironical and clownish postures, a disguised rebellion against orthodox physicians.

The practices of these charlatans must be compared, before being condemned, with the condition of medicine in the society in which they lived. If there had been less dishonesty and arrogance on the part of medical doctors, there would have been less opportunity for fraud on the part of charlatans. It must not be forgotten that among these maligned quacks were valuable empirics and skilled healers who for centuries were the only hope, the only comfort, for the masses deprived of any sort of care or assistance. Often the trappings of these "humbug vendors" concealed spirits in defiance against a medical hierarchy that was unable not only to provide a cure, but even to offer comfort.

Introduction:
The Toad and the Small Bird

One early October morning in 1922, a rickety ambulance locally known as the "loon catcher," haphazardly painted gray, with barred windows and a mattress-lined interior, began its careful descent down the steep bends that lead from the town of Volterra to the plain. The two robust attendants from the Royal Insane Asylum had been given orders to apprehend, in the town of C. M., a patient afflicted with an "acute crisis of delirious paranoia": a dangerous lunatic for whom a straitjacket had been provided, as dictated by the rules of procedure.

The ambulance, its engine steaming after a strenuous trip over rocky roads, finally came to a halt in the main square of the town. There an unforeseeable turn of events confronted the two attendants from the mental hospital. The local policeman who was to escort them to the patient informed them in somewhat embarrassed tones that this would not be possible, for the man could no longer be found; he had disappeared, vanished into thin air. The policeman expressed himself awkwardly, explaining that the "presumed madman" had no fixed abode in the town and only appeared from time to time. He declared that he knew the man personally and could guarantee that although a bit eccentric, he was certainly not crazed enough to be shut up in an asylum. Expressing sincere regret for the inconvenience, he advised the two men to get back in their ambulance and return to the hospital.

After their initial surprise, the dumbfounded attendants decided that the tale was totally implausible; they suspected that the lunatic had been hidden, a doubt confirmed by the presence of a group of curious onlookers, who commented on the policeman's words with a mocking and amused air. A furious dispute broke out, and by the time the "loon catcher" had started on its way back, the policeman and the inhabitants of the village had been covered with a deluge of oaths, insults and threats by the frustrated attendants, immediately requited with words of derision, laughter, and vulgar sounds of scorn.

The tale, embroidered with colorful and amusing variations, made the rounds of the nearby villages. After a time, a rumor spread that the man who had been saved from the mental hospital had run away to his native town in the distant south, and the episode was forgotten. But the feigned madman was actually still present: Expert at dissimulation and fraud, he had succeeded in deceiving not only the authorities who had drawn up the certificate of insanity, but also those who knew him well. This masquerade was not very difficult for an itinerant actor, a quack and merchant of remedies who for years had performed in the village squares, selling his wares to the public using ability, wit and guile.

His sudden attacks of insanity had strangely begun to occur soon after the mayor of the town had decided to put an end to what he considered a "public embarrassment" by denouncing the charlatan for illegal practice of the medical profession. From that moment on, in order to evade the law and continue his trade undisturbed, the quack had faded from sight. Although he no longer appeared in public, the simple people of the villages and the countryside knew where to find him, knew where to ask for and listen to his advice, how to obtain his remedies and follow his cures. Nothing could obscure the fame that he had acquired in the many years since he had left his Sicilian village to wander throughout the country with his painted cart overflowing with medicinal goods, performing at fairs or in the markets, assuring with his powerful barker's voice that he could provide remedies that would cure all ills, from tuberculosis to scabies, from headache to worms, and that he could soothe any sort of pain by virtue of the mysterious electrical effluvia that Mother Nature had kindly entrusted to his hands.

More than eighty years have passed, but the tale of the contest between this eccentric charlatan and a young man who had come to that isolated town to begin his career as a country doctor is part of the distant memories that remain with me from my childhood. My father was then fresh out of medical school, confronting his first demanding professional experience; he was full of enthusiasm, with absolute faith in the infallibility of his scientific knowledge — in those times a rather modest package of notions, on a par with the few instruments of his profession, jealously guarded in his inseparable black bag.

The village where he began his practice was an ancient Tuscan ham-

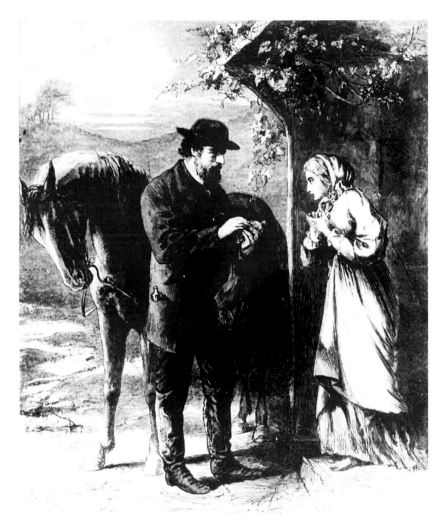

"A Country Doctor," A. R. Ward, 1869. U.S. National Library of Medicine, Bethesda, MD.

let clinging to the top of a small mountain, with dark stone houses huddled against one another as if for protection, separated by narrow, dark lanes that unexpectedly opened onto luminous, windswept archways through which could be viewed a distant, glittering sea.

To choose a practice in a place so isolated and poor was a question of vocation, a personal preference for a life of sacrifice and self-denial. No one at the time — least of all the person concerned — expected that the doctor of such a town would become rich: A six-thousand-lira stipend a year plus an allowance for his horse was all that he could expect, for almost the entire population, as the announcement for the competition had clearly stated, was on the official list of the indigent. His reward, therefore, if any, would have to be sought in the prestige, in the respect and gratitude of those he would help, and sometimes, with the aid of his knowledge, cure.

For a physician with little or no experience, a diagnosis was often a difficult enigma to decipher. He had to depend essentially on his own intuition; he performed the few laboratory tests, whose number could be counted on the fingers of one hand, with the help of a small microscope, a centrifuge, and some test tubes. When faced with a more difficult case, he wondered what use it was to spend such effort in recognizing a disease that he did not have the means to cure. The problems that besieged him were tuberculosis, pneumonia, typhus, diphtheria, the quaking fevers of malaria. He knew about microbes, which he considered his personal enemies, but he had no way to combat them; any neglected wound, even the most insignificant, could easily become a dreaded erysipelas or a fatal septicemia.

Although he expected all these difficulties, he had no idea that he had come to a town where, years before his arrival, a skillful charlatan had managed to acquire the reputation of a thaumaturge, or miracle worker, by performing impossible healings that the recipients of his aid still recounted during night vigils. Gradually, the young doctor came to realize that another form of occult and potent medicine was being practiced alongside his own by an ignorant lout who cured illnesses without knowing the secrets of the body, without need of any diagnostic certainty.

The first testimony to the ability of this crafty rogue was offered by the parish priest, a poor ecclesiastic garbed in a threadbare habit studded with patches and stains, who during the terrible Spanish influenza had conducted more funerals than baptisms and marriages. In the midst of this divine scourge, the charlatan had managed to earn a considerable amount of money selling, as a preventative against the contagion, little bottles containing "water from the Jordan," supposedly transported from the Holy Land.

More detailed and disturbing information was provided by the pharmacist, a little old man with a face as wrinkled as a turtle's. In the back room of his small pharmacy, he transformed into real substances the prescriptions written by my father, full of mysterious abbreviations: "sic jubeo" or "fiat lege artis." As the pharmacist crushed in his mortar the bitter powders that customers would swallow wrapped in wafers, he continuously complained about the innumerable herbal mixtures and other rubbish that the quack offered at inexpensive prices: dangerous concoctions that were more popular than his own, prepared according to the exacting standards of the true pharmacopoeia. The pharmacist's earnings had dropped considerably; few customers seemed tempted to buy the latest specialties advertised by smiling, satisfied faces in the yellowed pictures displayed in his window.

In the early days of his practice, the doctor noticed that his patients often behaved strangely: They appreciated his skill and courage in stopping a hemorrhage or assisting at a difficult birth, but they balked when it came to following his therapeutic prescriptions. Next to their beds he often discovered colored bottles full of unknown mixtures; when he reproached his patients, he received vague, hesitant answers. He resolved to fight the quack's outrageous pretenses and false remedies with his own rational, scientific knowledge.

Some years later an extraordinary incident occurred. A young grammar school teacher, the widow of a lieutenant immortalized on the memorial to the war's dead, was stricken by a grave pulmonary infection, a diffused pneumonia of uncertain nature, with a strange and inexplicable course. From the beginning the case was recognized as extremely serious. The doctor tried every cure, every possible remedy, but in vain. A renowned physician, called as consultant, was pessimistic; just as he was leaving, he spoke through the lowered window of his big black automobile, advising, as a final effort, an experimental new therapy involving injections of milk serum, which he instructed the doctor to sterilize by boiling in his small surgery. But the new therapy had no effect, and it seemed as though the gentle girl's breath was being slowly snuffed out, almost as if she were dying of love, mourned by the entire populace.

During one of his evening visits the doctor had a disturbing encounter, the only time that he and the charlatan ever met: Coming out the door, a thin man with an angular, lined face, wrapped in a green cape, cast him a baleful, taunting glance before disappearing into the dark. In the dim and silent atmosphere of the sickroom, someone was giving the patient a smoking greenish potion; beside the bed a toad struggled, crucified on two crossed reeds; from a beam overhead hung a cage with a small, hopping bird.

Indignant and offended, the doctor berated the relatives, who defended themselves by confessing that this was a last, desperate attempt to save the young woman. They admitted that the charlatan had been visiting secretly for days, comforting her and assuring her that she would soon regain her health. According to his words, the sick woman was "scorched inside," incapable of recovery, like a spider trapped in its own web. They had been told to abandon the medical remedies that had been proven useless and entrust her to his care. Nothing could make them change their irrational decision, not even the doctor's threat of abandonment, nor his words of derision and scorn for their ignorance and for the danger of their choice. Long days went by, and the townspeople waited with bated breath; then, inexplicably, a slow and progressive improvement began, followed by a complete recovery, which everyone, obviously, attributed to the charlatan's magical therapy.

The young doctor, considering himself the loser, meditated on this incident, one of many that he judged personal defeats. Confronted by his failures, he tried to understand the cunning maneuvers of the elusive, mysterious individual who challenged him with his irrational methods. He wondered what possible real curative powers could be possessed by a coarse, ignorant merchant of remedies over whose head hung the condemnation of the law. Did the secret of his success depend on luck, magic, personal magnetism, or simply a contemptible and treacherous suggestion? At the same time, the doctor began to feel less secure in his vigorous defense of science, in his insistence that all of the charlatan's methods were despicably fraudulent. In spite of himself, he had to admit that in some cases the mystifications, the abstruse and fantastic therapies could obtain unexpected results, effects that lay outside the field of any logical explanation. He began to believe not only that the process of healing required the remedies of orthodox medicine, but that other mysterious elements could mediate the course of a disease. He suspected that he would have to search for the cause of his failures in himself, in his behavior as an objective healer, scrupulous in his scientific honesty but incapable of expressing intimacy, comfort, empathy.

When he had placed his ear to his patient's chest, he had not heard her inner voices; he had forsaken her, left her in a state of desolate despair, incapable of fighting her illness, resigned to an unconscious self-destruction. The person who had appeared as a comforting, consoling magician had offered her a different remedy, sacred and mystical. The doctor was now able to grasp the meaning of that ridiculous scene: The ugly dying toad was the symbol of the regressing malady; the bird indicated the return of hope in the fullness of life. He saw that the charlatan, with his suggestive art, had merely given the patient a chance to believe in what she herself wished to believe. His shadowy, arcane practices had succeeded in influencing her spirit and her feelings, had spurred her to call on the mysterious curative powers of her own reaction to the disease, the only true natural processes that could lead to recovery.

More than twenty years passed, and in those twenty years the science of medicine achieved goals more prodigious than any attained in the preceding twenty centuries. The young country doctor, now a skilled practitioner, realized with surprise that all the marvelous technical and scientific apparatus that he now had access to had not completely succeeded in replacing the medicine of herbs and mysteries. Other heretical practices, other illicit healers, other superstitions had emerged to challenge official medicine, to win the minds of the public: Ancient, irrational cures, toward which his colleagues displayed derision or a visceral disdain, managed to fill each gap left open by medicine's every weakness, every uncertainty.

All around him, countless specialists serving in the ranks of collective medicine were repeating his early mistakes; it was easier, safer, more convenient for them to act simply as technicians, as interpreters of scientific precepts, rather than be truly involved with an ailing patient by transforming themselves, through their acts and words, into healers. It became apparent to him that quackery was not merely a reprehensible fraud but also a fascinating phenomenon intimately entwined with human nature: a phenomenon whose relationship with curing had been indissoluble since the origins of medicine, a form of the art of healing which had risen by necessity out of popular empiricism and that had to be thoroughly understood before being judged.

He remembered the lesson he had learned from the charlatan in the difficult years of his youth: Any endeavor to heal had a greater chance of success if it included a sympathetic dimension of hope, compassion, and support, if an intimate bond between healer and patient could be created. The wily charlatan no longer seemed merely a despicable impostor; somehow, with his symbolic gestures deprived of any logic he had succeeded in arousing the mysterious healing forces of nature and had answered an irrepressible human need. Unconsciously, in his deception, he had behaved like a primitive psychotherapist.

Ma chi vuole raccontare tutti i modi, e tutte le maniere che adoperano i ciarlatani per fare bezzi, havrà da fare assai.

"But he who wishes to recount all the methods, and all the deceits that charlatans use to gain money, will have much to do."

Thomas Garzoni da Bagnocavallo, Lateran canon, in
La Piazza Universale di Tutte le Professioni del Mondo

CHAPTER 1

"People who go about swindling, with little exertion and for their own gain"

Charlatans in the Middle Ages and Beyond

Ever since medieval times, the lowliest charlatans, who sold balms and herbal mixtures, juleps, quintessences, stones, amulets, and every sort of miraculous medicinal secret, mingled with an endless crowd of vagrants. The overwhelming majority of these popular vendors never acquired any refinement of manner or success; they were small-time peddlers, impoverished vagabonds confused amongst a rabble of thieves, beggars, and idlers who went from tavern to tavern in the countryside and the villages, living off any expedient that would allow them to eat, associating with those "who go wandering through the World, and have no fixed Seat or firm Habitation in any place." Thus, with ill-concealed disdain, Marc'Antonio Savelli of Modigliana describes them in his "Universal Practice," a work that he himself calls "most lofty and necessary to persons of every rank." The harsh censor indicates how difficult it was to keep out of the cities and countryside of the Florentine dominion all these persons who "go around swindling in order not to work," a troublesome, ceaselessly wandering mass made up of "bilkers, blackguards, beggars, paupers, bogus sick, mendicants, gypsies, and counterfeiters of every type." Among this ragged crew roamed "mountebanks, quacks and charlatans," all dedicated to "deceiving people by acting as doctors."[1]

Popular charlatans drifted from place to place, living hand to mouth, sleeping in inns or in haylofts, or accepting the hospitality of some peasant, whom they repaid with an ointment or a prodigious elixir. Taverns were generally the preferred, if not the obligatory, stopping place of those who had no definite home; there they met other outcasts such as prostitutes, disbanded soldiers, cardsharps, small-time tricksters, and vagabonds of every sort.

Scipione Mercuri, the Dominican Friar Jerome, was a man who had lived an adventurous life; he was fond of introducing himself in his writings as "philosopher, doctor, and Roman Citizen"; a cleric with the "beard of a doctor and the tonsure of a priest," ardent supporter of the caste of erudite physicians to which, with pride, he belonged. Endowed with a passionate and polemical disposition, he did not hesitate to upbraid these false doctors, knaves whom he branded with stinging phrases, recalling that Saint Thomas had said, "One cannot listen to a Charlatan without fear of mortal sin." He put the gullible populace on their guard, reminding them that when the comedy is over, the charlatan relaxes at the inn "and at table among his Buffoons, carouses and laughs in the faces of those fools" whose money he has taken. The friar could not comprehend why people bought the remedies of frauds "with more faith than they do those prescribed by doctors, the foolish public assuming that a vagabond and frequenter of taverns knows better, having studied in no other book than that of the whore."

The sale of medical remedies was often combined with the offer of baubles and cosmetics; it was a way to make ends meet and have a valid alibi ready for any suspicious bailiff who patrolled the squares by order of the College of Physicians. "For your own good," Mercuri admonishes charlatans, "it is time that you stop practicing the sublime subject of medicine"; he counsels them to limit their sales to "trinkets, such as soaps, creams, sacred images, rings against the evil eye, pleasant stories, powders for whitening the teeth, paste for calluses."[2]

A century later, in a collection of seventeenth-century "Amiable Venetian Satires," the academician Sebastiano Rossi scornfully asks charlatans, "Why are you always so miserable and such fools?" If you are so eloquent, if you can charm snakes, if you are successful at selling "fake unguents and other rubbish," how is it that you do not even have "shoes on your feet?"[3]

Various Charlatans, Various Trades

Who is a charlatan: a despicable vagabond, a "wretch in fancy dress," an innocuous blabbermouth who for profit or vanity pretends medical knowledge that he does not possess? Or only a fool, a jester who uses his show to palm off miraculous remedies on an ignorant and naive audience? Or rather a malicious merchant, who beneath the disguise of a healer, manages to poison people with his false cures, a treacherous individual that Professor Tissot, illustrious Swiss academic and physician of Voltaire, considered more dangerous than a vulgar highway assassin?

The "Vocabulary" compiled by the Academy of the Crusca, a literary association founded in Florence in 1582 for the purpose of purifying the Tuscan language, describes a charlatan as "one who peddles unguents and other medicines, pulls teeth, and also does conjuring tricks in the public square": a poor quack who, to market his products, resorts to clowning, recitation, acrobatics, singing, sleight of hand, and fantastic tricks. The Italian verb "ciarlare," means to make useless and long-winded speeches, chatter in a tiresome and vain manner, talk nonsense; it is an onomatopoeic verb that seems to "wed the sound of the cicada to idle speech."

The Italian language has many names to distinguish quacks according to their specialized behavior. "Cerretano" is the oldest Italian epithet: In the beginning it did not refer only to vendors of ointments and medicines, but generically indicated a mass of deceivers who, in the Middle Ages, devoted themselves to "rapacious begging." The name "cerretano" came from the Umbrian town of Cerreto: Flavio Biondo, in "Italia Illustrata," published in 1474, wrote: "Between the steep and Barren mountains of Umbria rises Cerreto, Castle of recent name, and abounding with inhabitants; and from this castle are named Cerretani, those who go wandering all over Italy with different customs, under different colors, and with different deceits for the purpose of digging money from the pockets of their fellowmen." In the fifteenth century, Teseo Pini, an inflexible vicar and ecclesiastical judge, "expertus in Truffis," was charged with the suppression of this "plague" from Cerreto; he lists the range of their activities: "false doctors, false hermits, false preachers, fabricators of false reliquaries, false enchanters, false soothsayers, trappers (who catch gulls), rascals, cheaters and mendicants."[4]

Saint Antoninus, archbishop of Modena in the fourteenth century, indignantly noted that all of these hypocritical simulators travel around "to acquire rich and plentiful alms without having much need under the guise of just and good inhabitants of Cerreto." In short, a motley crowd of rascals who "deceive men sullying the name of the honest people of this pleasant town." Pope Innocent VIII even called for a crusade, ordering Brother Bernard of Feltre to dispatch a mission against these frauds from Cerreto "pessimum et fraudolentum hominum genius." Other "wandering rascals" emerged from this gallery of cheats, who pretended to be herbalists, doctors, and alchemists. The names "cerretano" and "ciarlatano" began to have the same meaning toward the end of the sixteenth century and referred almost always to those extravagant personages who peddled popular medicines in the square.[5]

Over time, the designation "charlatan" acquired a broader and more ambiguous meaning: In addition to the salesman of remedies and trinkets or the successful quack, it came to include the histrionic necromancer, the empirical herbalist, the false alchemist, and the pseudoscientist. In addition, many traveling surgeons who worked in various specialties, without either license or training, were included by right into the family of charlatans, so that distinguishing the skilled healer in good faith from the callous and inept fraud was often an arduous task.

"Charlatan" was soon adopted by all the European countries; "charlatan" has remained in the French language even after futile endeavors to deny its Italian origin; there was an attempt to link the word to a certain Dr. Latan, who rode about the streets of Paris in a cart, searching out the sick, selling medicines for every ailment. He was so famous that as soon as the common folk spied him from afar they would cry, "Voilà le char de Latan." The distortion "ciarlatini," indicating charlatans of foreign origin, is sometimes found in English texts. Around the sixteenth century, English-speaking countries adopted the word "quack" and defined every charlatanesque activity as "quackery." A popular, nineteenth-century verse was: "A potent quack long versed in human ills, who first insults the victims whom he kills." "Quack quack" sounds like the petulant squawking of a goose, a duck, a barnyard fowl. It resembles the Sicilian "quaquaraquà," synonym for a lower-level subordinate who prattles constantly in the hopes of seeming more important than he really is.

In paintings, as in numerous satirical drawings and prints, the charlatan is depicted as he operates from atop a platform in the square; it was necessary for him to be elevated not only to present his merchandise, but also so that his voice could be better heard by all; to stand on a platform implicated supremacy, skill, culture, a means by which to better dominate the public. The common name of "mountebank" was derived from "montare in banco," to climb onto a stand. A ban posted in 1571, conserved in the archives of the Kingdom of Naples, announces: "Surmis'd, the great abundance of Charlatans who come to this most faithful city of Naples … it is ordered that no Charlatan, or Mountebank … dare, or presume, from this day forward, and as long as this Lent will last, mount on a platform to harangue, or sell ointments, oils, soaps & other things, nor images or rosaries, before day past nineteen hours [around twelve noon], and the same when Lent has passed, on Sunday and Feast day, under pain of four strappado, to be carried out irrevocably, or other punishment reserved to the judgment of this Grand Court. All beware of contravention."[6]

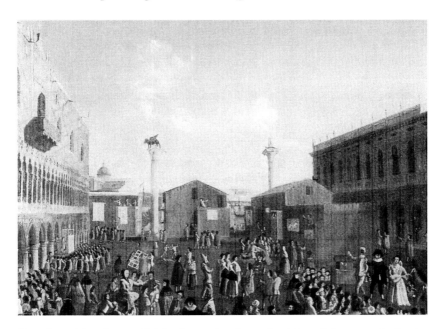

"Ciarlatani in Piazzetta" (Charlatans in Piazza San Marco) from a painting by Gabriel Bella. Fondazione Querini Stampaglia Venice (1750).

Fynes Moryson, an attentive, seventeenth-century English traveler, described the hordes of empirics who went from one market square to the next. They were called mountebanks because they stood on benches or stages to sell their wares; to attract a larger crowd, they hired a Zany, or masked buffoon, and sometimes a woman. The audience threw them money wrapped in handkerchiefs, which they returned with their products, usually distilled waters, or the more popular ointments to soothe pain or cure scabies.[7]

"Saltimbanco" was a name reserved for those who "accepted a reward for giving delight": jugglers, wandering tumblers, who in order to sell remedies performed public exhibitions of dexterity and skill. Physical ability was very much appreciated by the public: "My hand is quicker than my brain," cried Della Pergola from his bench; this charlatan knew that his public was attracted more by his skill as a conjurer than by his chatter. He traveled from fair to fair at the end of the eighteenth century, his curious motto serving to summon the crowds: On his table were cards, balls and cones which he used like any modern magician. A characteristic of the saltimbanco was his habit of working alone without a real company; theirs was an ancient art, inherited from the funambulists of Roman times.

Sometimes the Latin word "circulator" can be found in judicial proceedings, a name used to brand individuals as rogues with an "anima naturaliter circulatoria," a term that underlines their incessant wandering in the most disparate localities. "Circumforaneus" or "circulatores" were in fact the names with which the Romans designated lazy time wasters.

The Lateran canon Thomaso Garzoni da Bagnocavallo describes all these quacks in action: "On all sides one sees the square filled with these charlatans; some sell powder to reduce flatulence from behind.... [S]ome propose Philosopher's Oil as the quintessence for getting rich; some sell mullein oil for colds, or an ointment made from the fat of a gelding for hernias, or an unguent for scabies that improves the memory, or cat or dog feces as a poultice for hernias.... [S]ome sell iron trusses for broken bones, some slaked-lime paste for killing mice." Others demonstrate a series of fantastic gimmicks, offering "eyeglasses to see in the dark," perhaps in anticipation of infrared spectacles, or, like circus ringmasters, "show dreadful monsters, horrifying to contemplate." Illusionists perform magic tricks: One "washes his face with liquid lead," another pretends to cut off someone's nose with an artificial knife, while a third tries out the trivial joke of convincing a person to eat excrement disguised as a tasty mouthful.[8]

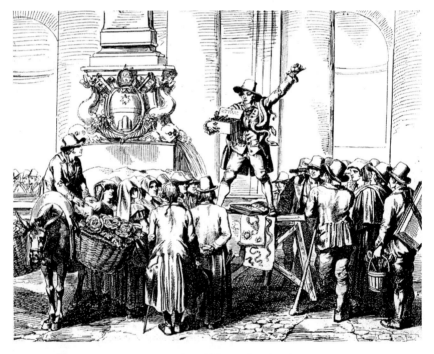

A charlatan in Rome, a viper on his shoulder, promises health. Acquaforte by B. Pinelli, Roma, 1821. Biblioteca Nazionale Centrale, Firenze.

The philosopher Benedetto Croce, in "The Neapolitan Theater," describes a type of charlatan called "ciaravole" or "ciaraldo" who went around with a box of snakes, performing in shows, playing games and selling poultices; others performed "bagattelle" or "guarattelle," demonstrations of deftness; still others used marionettes to improvise lively comedies.[9]

Popular charlatans blended with other kinds of peddlers, and even with water sellers, or with vendors of sweets and various spices, for there was often an undefinable connection between these delicacies and the charlatans' medicines, made with sugar and alcohol, which, even if ineffective, were at least pleasing to the taste.

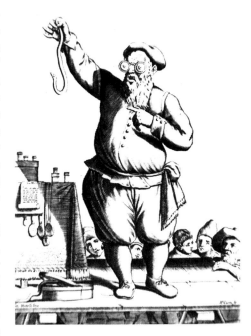

"The Charlatan and the Snake" Satirical engraving by G.M. Mitelli (1760). The charlatan wears thick lenses so as to appear a man of science and does not fear the snake's bite. Biblioteca Nazionale Centrale, Firenze.

Licenses for Charlatans: The Carrot and the Stick

Scipione Mercuri considered charlatans to be "vagabonds, perjurers, blabbermouths, whoremongers, cardsharps ... and refined liars." If what they promised were true, "they would not have to go constantly wandering, roving from inn to inn, nor stopping in the Cities." If only one of the remedies that they sold possessed the virtues that they so persistently proclaim, "it would be enough to make them rich."[10]

But Mercuri, blinded by irrepressible disdain, was not always correct; in fact, the designation "charlatan" had not always been derogatory, nor did it possess the meaning that it acquired in later times. The small-time, modest merchants who manufactured and sold, under license by the medical authorities, unguents, balsams, poultices, oils, colyrium and herbal compositions made with medicinal plants were also called charlatans, an authorization that can be traced to a time in which an attempt was made to define the role of every healer. In order to protect his subjects from "imperitia medicorum," the enlightened monarch Roger II, king of Sicily, issued a decree in 1134, threatening severe punishment, "carceri constringatur," and confiscation of property for anyone who practiced medicine without the permission of the officials and judges. Later, his grandson Frederick II issued decrees that at least in theory were meant to do away with the activity of illegal practitioners. The first edicts banning the illegal practice of medicine, with strict penalties for transgressors, were published during his reign. Doctors in medicine, the "physici" who graduated from the first schools, were thus qualified; at the same time an endeavor was made to create a clear and insuperable barrier between orthodox medicine and illegal practice. The celebrated School of Salerno undertook the task of seriously organizing skilled healers, experienced practitioners, bringing them under the jurisdiction of the civic authorities, but often patients preferred illegitimate healers to the official doctors, and quackery, chased out of the front door, came back in through the window.

When the Colleges of Physicians were established, the possibility of obtaining a precise role in the ranks of the health administration arrived at last even for charlatans. At the beginning of the fifteenth century these colleges acted as tribunals that decided affairs dealing with public health. In order to keep all illegal practitioners under control, from the empirical peddler of mixtures made from plants to the charlatan who performed in the squares, the authorities adopted the rule of the carrot and the stick: If these individuals did not submit to the health authorities they became outlaws, to be persecuted and condemned. In the archives of every historical city in Italy there are numerous documents that reveal how charlatans, in order to become recognized and practice without running into trouble, had to apply to the colleges, declare the composition of their "secrets," demonstrate the nature of the substances that they used and explain to the examiners how they intended to make their preparations: a long, bureaucratic procedure, intended less as an attempt to protect the peoples' health than as a demonstration of the authority of physicians and apothecaries, a precaution necessary to defend the professional monopoly of their powerful corporations from the competition of these able merchants.

In medieval Florence a practitioner was not qualified by doctoral titles alone; an empiric, even if by profession a shoemaker, once he was judged able to remove a cataract, could be inscribed in the guild along with the doctor that held a diploma from Padua. At the beginning of the fifteenth century, the College of Palermo authorized special licenses for some practitioners who had no title; most were chosen with regard solely for their empirical experience: A practitioner was authorized to cure broken bones or was specialized in "restoring dislocated limbs"; another was assigned to curing abscesses of the testicles or extracting bladder stones.[11]

Examples of these licenses, the so-called privileges or matriculas, issued to charlatans, often transcribed with uncertain spelling by the registrars, can be found in the proceedings of the College of Physicians in Siena: a moving testimony that records an uninterrupted procession of charlatans of lowly rank appearing before the examiners in an arc of nearly three centuries; an anonymous crowd attempting to make up for the modesty of their condition by offering medicines with grandiloquent, evocative names like "Oil of the Sun," "Claw of the Great Beast," "Spirit of Gold," "Tooth of the Sea Dog," "Treasure of Health," "Cloth of Well Being," "Oil of the Madonna," and innumerable "Elixirs of Long Life." These remedies, by virtue of their name alone, were supposed to intrigue and seduce the public. The examiners were advised to be particularly attentive and strict in controlling the substances that the charlatans intended to sell, given their reputation for being "not very respectable people, full of falsehoods and lies."[12]

In choosing their own nicknames the charlatans preferred instead to adopt sobriquets of a popular stamp, decidedly humbler than the fancy names attached to their remedies. Presenting themselves before the examiners at the college were the "Little Bourgeois," "the Faithful One," the "Golden Forehead," the "Maltese," the "Iron Leg," the "Peasant": simple folk trying to make ends meet, who appeared with good-natured cheer, as if to excuse the inevitable deception concealed in their miraculous therapies. These were colleagues and rivals of other wandering quacks who journeyed through the towns of Italy, like "Johnny the Bolognese," the "Greengrocer," the "Little American," "Pulcinello," and even a "National Idiot." An odd or humorous nickname might even serve to attract the sympathy of the public.[13]

Carlo Francesco Sarri peddled "The Spaniard's Oil," along with breath-sweetening lozenges made of a remarkable paste whose composition, the charlatan claimed, was a secret given him by a noble and mysterious lady.

Gian Francesco Rossi presented "Oil of the Sun," an "illuminating and life-giving" remedy. This time the examiners were suspicious of the charlatan and stubbornly insisted on knowing the type of "manipulation" and the nature of the substances he had used, even though it was a harmless herbal mixture made of rue, rosemary, plantain, mountain sage, storax "tears" or resin, with the addition of incense and oil of turpentine: a soothing recipe for the respiratory paths that could honorably figure among a modern herbalist's prescriptions.

One stratagem often used by charlatans to obtain a favorable judgment from the College of Physicians was to include in the list of remedies one or more substances that figured in the rich official pharmacopoeia; the examiners could not reject elements that they themselves prescribed. Lorenzo Sabatini, a Roman charlatan, required permission to sell, as a cure for pneumonia and gout, his "Balm of Human Fat," a "useful and repercussive" ingredient "for pain of the nerves" that could be found in various compositions commonly used in official therapy. In order to be effective, this fat was supposed to come from a healthy man, killed in an accident or for exemplary punishment, and its cost was prohibitive. In the case in question, with all probability the charlatan had simply slaughtered a pig.

Siena was one of the principal bridges between Western civilization and that of the East, and many of the familiar emblems associated with the city could be traced to the sacred symbols of Asia.[14] The Sienese public was particularly fascinated by drugs with exotic names, brought by intrepid travelers from the faraway Orient. Obviously, many of these remedies, promoted as coming from India and China, were simple homemade preparations. In the year 1735 there was an unusual number of requests to the College of Physicians of Siena from various "foreign" charlatans, who offered precious "arcanums," possessing extraordinary medicinal properties, that they had discovered during their imaginary voyages. An individual who qualified himself as the "Italian Charlatan Operator" offered his prodigious "Egyptian Balm," but had to compete with a rival, who, to validate the genuineness of his "Arabian Balm," presented himself as a "Turk become Christian"; "at least this is in accordance with what he declared," the perplexed clerk noted, after having contemplated the face of the improbable Turk.

Another "Oriental Balm" was presented in 1779 by Pietro Barbarini, a charlatan from Portoferraio on the island of Elba. This time, at the bottom of the file is a singular footnote in his favor, written in the hand of the chief physician. This influential personage suggests that since the charlatan is "an unfortunate wretch, it would be of sentiment to concede the permit with very small expense," renouncing his own fee, and at once imitated by the other two counselors.[15] A gesture of such extraordinary generosity would have been difficult to obtain in other cities, given the tormented and stormy relations between medical authorities and charlatans.

Another example of benevolence toward charlatans can be read in a permit granted on October 30, 1717. "Silvestro Camisciano, Charlatan of Sicily presenting himself to the College, requested license to sell the Balm called *Oriental* and other." The noble college, after examining the recipes of his compositions, gives its approval and "concedes the Privilege in Parchment according to his request," an exceedingly magnanimous concession, as parchment was reserved for the licenses and diplomas of practitioners of superior rank.[16]

An expedient sometimes used to obtain a license for a particular remedy was to include in its ingredients those with a sacred or sanctimonious name. An ointment brought before the examiners by a charlatan from Pistoia had the venerable label of "Manus Dei" and was approved without difficulty; in 1724, another vagabond presented his "Innocent Balm," a miraculous mixture that was supposed to function in virtue of the "Holy memory of Pope Innocent the Eleventh."

The charlatans who arrived from the southern states of Italy were even shrewder. Aniello Landolfi, under the pseudonym "The Great Neapolitan," listed the merits of a prodigious medicine that he had prepared with rue, anise, and juniper. He confidently promised that four drops on the chest and on the spine were sufficient to "transmit by imperceptible transpiration" the malignant humors, thus purifying the blood and destroying bile; the mere odor alone forces worms to abandon the bodies of children and protects against apoplexy.

Francesco Fasano came from the "Land of Basilicata" with a document attesting the esteem in which he was held by His Majesty, the King of the Two Sicilies, a document which had been without doubt fashioned by the charlatan himself but which the excellent doctors of Siena were forced to consider. His remedy was an insuperable collyrium "for the eyes and their infirmities," made from verbena, rosemary blossoms, celandine and cloves, mixed with honey and white wine and even with Congo pepper; happily for the user, he advised its application "in a tender amount."

A Bullying Hierarchy

The charlatan Gaetano de Milan presented himself to his numerous admirers claiming to be a famous thaumaturge, an "illustrious chemist and botanist of the Royal Academy of Paris" who was "engaged in the healing of the most difficult maladies and the cure of those given up for desperate by professors." Actually he was a former confectioner who had fled from his creditors and returned, at the end of the eighteenth century, to his native city, Milan. Regardless of his success with the public, the medical statutes of Milan, stricter than in other cities, often obliged him to leave town. De Milan spent his whole life escaping from the authorities, reappearing as soon as things quieted down. Finally, the chief physician of the college, exasperated by his insistent requests, granted de Milan entrance to the examinations. The two examining physicians judged him "incapable and ignorant, not being able to distinguish afflictions nor pen the formulae of the remedies." The charlatan claimed that this verdict was not because he was "lacking in Art," but because of his lowly birth, an assertion that was not entirely unlikely, for the position and wealth of the applicant's family were elements that could change the faculty's judgment. Resigned at last to the futility of his entreaties, he "humbly beseeches Your Excellency to order that he be given a passport for his safety, gratis, in order to go to Germany."[17]

The intention of taking a wife or the responsibility of providing for numerous offspring could sometimes be an effective ploy, used to move the authorities to pity. In 1630, Paulo Roneti, a charlatan nicknamed "Coccapane," returned with his small company of players to the Florentine Grand Duchy. This time the bailiffs refused to allow him to sell his remedies in the square with the excuse that his old license had expired. Coccapane suspected that since he was "A Jew become Christian," the main hindrance was his race, for the crowds were attracted by Jewish medicasters, believed to have inherited arcane practices from their ancestors; along with their incantations, steeped in magic and astrology, they often brought miraculous stones and strange herbs from the faraway Orient. Coccapane petitioned His Serene Highness, the Grand Duke Ferdinand, "with knees to the ground" that "for the love of God concede [the license] again so that he can mount his stand along with his company as before." If the license were granted, he would make two promises: the first, that he would remain in "the most holy Christian faith"; the second is even more singular: "[A]fterwards I shall wed."[18] The license was awarded, but the Grand Duke did not seem wholly convinced by the charlatan's matrimonial promise and added a footnote, written in his own hand: "Granted, but without women."

Even when a license was obtained, the charlatan was not allowed to use the remedies that he sold in any way except externally; they were not to be administered by mouth. The erudite physician alone was the authorized healer of internal ills, the sole person who could give out orders regarding diet and "universal evacuations." The mouth, an entrance jealously reserved for the medical concoctions of physicians, was shut tight for charlatans. This rigid limitation probably originated from ancient religious beliefs; the apertures of the body were entrances for poisonous and malignant spirits that carried every sort of disease and had to be jealously guarded. From the early Middle Ages it was believed that diseases carried by demons entered the body during sleep, through the mouth or the opposite orifice. It seems that Martin Luther, always counter to the mainstream, preferred to sleep with a naked bottom so that the demons could leave his body more easily.

In Sicily, as in other regions, ordinances charged with threats did not seem to prevent charlatans from administering medicines through the forbidden channel. In November of 1572, a prefect in Palermo admonished charlatans for the twentieth time not to "dispense any remedy or medicine taken by mouth."[19]

The examining physicians' incompetence in medical matters was often equal if not superior to that of the charlatans, therefore the judgment of the "expert" doctors regarding the remedies of quacks is somewhat bewildering. The lack of any academic title, and not their capacity as healers, was almost always the only possible distinction between doctors and charlatans. The mixtures offered by the charlatans, made from extracts of plants and herbs, were often superior in effectiveness to those prescribed by physicians. At the very least they were usually innocuous, simple in preparation, and, a fact not to be ignored, accessible to the meager purses of the populace. With the excuse of saving the population from hypothetical poisoning, the medical college sometimes obliged an unfortunate quack to swallow his concoctions in their presence; since these were usually unguents and balms composed of oily substances, it was decidedly unpleasant for the poor wretch.

If the examination had a positive outcome, after paying a tax the charlatan could obtain a privilege, or matricula, but only for a limited time. Once he had mounted his platform in the square, he could begin the sale of his remedies. Yet he remained on the bottom rung of the ladder of medical hierarchy, beneath the surgeons, the barbers, and the pig butchers, grudgingly tolerated and regarded with suspicion and mistrust by physicians and chemists. The fact that he had not followed any scholastic course, that he did not know a word of Latin or possess the slightest notion of philosophy or logic, and that he was totally ignorant of the canons of humoral medicine was manifest proof of his lowly and dangerous obscurantism. A common strategy used to combat charlatanism was founded on a demonstration of the quack's ignorance. Their empirical methods, whether beneficial or not, had to be condemned in any case because practiced by illiterate persons of lowly rank who could neither read nor write.

Broadsheets and Bans

A considerable number of charlatans chose to disobey the edicts and not pay any tax, as they considered the limitations placed on their universal cures unjust. Many of them never appeared before the College of Physicians and therefore enjoyed a freedom of action that the authorities would have either refused or severely restricted. They preferred to wander to places where it was easier to trade in all types of remedies, where they could express their own fantastic ideas, disregard the laws and practice the types of cures that were most congenial to them. The law provided stiff fines or even the arrest of these dangerous rebels who tolerated no restraints, and for habitual offenders, at least on paper, physical tortures such as strappado, lashes, or the stocks. These were all calculated risks, however, that were part of the hazards of their profession. Marc'Antonio Savelli warned that amongst these "vagabonds, and swindlers, deserving of every punishment, [there] are those who with false licenses and creeds go begging for the most part in the countryside, making simple persons believe all matter of things in order to take their money ... to cheat people, either behaving like Doctors, or similar." These "false doctors that go around the World selling medicinal secrets of no worth or professing to cure all, or many ills, cozening the simple not only of their money but often of their health and their life, must be punished with harsh penalties, according to the instances and the persons."[20]

It was no easy task for the medical authorities of the large cities to curtail the hordes of charlatans who gave proof of their operating skill before all eyes or sold secret mixtures that promised prodigious healings or renewed youth and beauty. But it was risky for those who had no license at all to sell their remedies if an indictment had been filed by a jealous physician or a furious apothecary. Then the bailiffs moved with unusual speed, proceeded to arrest the charlatan and dragged him to judgment. Deputies of the guards that acted as police for the College of Physicians had a standing order to seek out these "profit-eaters" that practiced everywhere without license.

By the end of the fifteenth century, the Florentine statutes threatened heavy fines for anyone who practiced medicine without a license; apothecaries were admonished not to deal with charlatans nor to lend them any sort of aid. To encourage delations, half of the fine provided for those who broke the law, "one hundred 'soldi' of small florins," was allotted to the person who made the secret accusation. Notwithstanding the interminable parade of bans and menacing edicts produced by the powerful medical colleges in every city, the number of charlatans in Italy grew constantly. Halfway through the sixteenth century Thomaso Garzoni anxiously noted: "[I]n our days the number, and the types of these people have grown like weeds, so that in every City, in every land, in every square one can see nothing other than Cerretani or Cantimbanchi. ... And all with various arts and frauds [they] delude the minds of the vulgar populace and entice their ears to listen to the lies they tell, their eyes to see the trifles, their senses to stand at attention for the ridiculous rehearsals that they make in the squares."[21]

The Grand Duchy of Tuscany spared no pity for this multitude of humble wanderers, the popular charlatans who roamed the countryside on foot, pulling all their pharmaceutical treasures and the boards for their stands on a miserable cart, branded with the reputation of "lazy and vice-ridden persons," who mingled with "vagabonds, scoundrels, gamblers, gypsies, [and] false beggars." A harsh edict ordered that "to prevent the occasion for people to uselessly dissipate themselves and to be deceived ... [f]or the future, all Charlatans, Mountebanks, Storytellers, Puppet-masters, Jugglers and all who show freaks of nature, Machines, Animals, or who sell secrets, or any other foreign person who wanders around earning his keep with a similar trade, are not to be permitted to stop in any City, Land, Castle or other place in the Grand Duchy to give spectacle, or to demonstrate their art or industry." A sole exception was granted to "country storytellers," of whom the populace were particularly fond, but before giving permission, it was to be ascertained "if, for their blindness, or other corporal imperfections these wanderers are otherwise unable to earn their living with another trade."[22]

In the Serene Republic of Venice, the incessant arrival of "lazy, pestering, and vagabond people," attracted by the riches of the splendid city, worried the authorities so much that from the fifteenth to the eighteenth centuries "terminations," or ordinances, were repeated with incessant monotony, commanding boatmen, under threat of dire penalty, not to ferry into the Venetian territories any "zarattani (charlatans), foreign beggars," capable of every fraud, who attempted any means to worm money out of their fellowmen. A petition was sent to the doge on May 20, 1603, by the priors and the College of Physicians and Apothecaries, stating that "many charlatans, dispersing themselves like refugees here and there, dupe the ignorant common people, professing to have particular secrets that benefit the human body, and having obtained licenses to trade, dispense one thing for another, cheating the people and causing infinite harm."[23] As if this were not enough, "many women indifferently order purging medications, and do all that one expects a learned and experienced physician to do." Friars, who feel protected by their condition, are amongst these illegal healers and others who "under cover of religion make witchcraft, giving violent medications to chase out spirits, and instead of chasing out the devil, for the most part chase out the soul."[24]

An ordinance issued on June 27, 1713, directed to the Venetian "Illustrious and Excellent Sires of the Highest Superintendence of Health," warns of the harm that could derive "to the Health of Subjects through the recklessness of Charlatans, greedy people intent only on pressing the Subjects with the wind of their voices, rather than with the virtues and knowledge of their substances."[25]

Hoping to evade the bans, charlatans did their utmost to obtain letters and credentials from important figures; if accused or captured, they pretended to be sincerely repentant, and did everything in their power to obtain a pardon. Some haughtily impugned the sentences of the judges with every captious objection, or sent endless pleas to the authorities, who, fed up in the end, let them go. In extreme cases a rapid escape became the best way to avoid a dangerous situation.

In reality, the innumerable edicts against charlatans, ploddingly repeated in every age and in every Italian state, only rarely, if at all, obtained the desired effect; quackery, which had found in Italy a warm welcome and a fertile terrain for its growth, by now had solidly planted its roots. The art of getting along in any situation, still evident today in Italians, gave birth to a myriad of extravagant personalities, who put to good use their inexhaustible imagination and subtle grandiloquence.

A close alliance united physicians and men of law. The founder of forensic medicine, the Sicilian Paolo Zacchia, believed that anyone who sold medical remedies should be condemned without hesitation. The reason was simple: Anyone who treats an unknown disease without knowing its cause falls into mortal sin; the illustrious judge did not take into consideration that this was valid not only for charlatans, but also for the entire medical class of his time.

Another judge of the seventeenth century, Antonio Maria Cospi, considered himself an unrivaled expert at detecting fraud and discovering the ubiquitous, unlicensed rascals. He gives infallible advice for unmasking these "impostors who go around in the world selling medicinal secrets, not only for many ills, but for all ills, cheating simple men and taking away not only their faculties but their lives, worthy in truth of mighty punishments." He explains how to discover their deceits, starting with a rigorous corporeal examination, not unlike that used today on criminals as they enter a maximum security prison: "[F]irst of all, he will be made to stand with his arms wide open," so that he cannot hide anything in his sleeves. He should then be stripped and reclothed with "other garb prepared by the judge." After a careful scientific evaluation regarding the color and the odor of all the confiscated medicines, the final judgment consists of a theoretical examination in the presence of experts, who should ask where "the malign humour resides in particular, if in the viscera or in the blood ...

and why he would apply these medicaments." And still taking into account the opinion of the experts, the judge shall inquire if this false doctor is "understanding of the art of medicine or not," and if someone had "received any harm to his life" or had been killed through his fault.[26]

A Benevolent Trial

For centuries, the city of Siena had been a fertile and coveted terrain, the preferred destination of wandering charlatans who arrived there in crowds, especially from the southern regions of Italy.

The College of Physicians of Siena, which functioned as a court of law for sanitary matters, was made up of only three counselors directed by a chief physician. The impression given is that of an assemblage of good people who raised their voices out of duty but rarely applied the strict penalties that were established by the law. The intransigence of the college toward charlatans and practitioners, considered a "phalanx of impostors, of quacks, of persons who took advantage of the simplemindedness of their fellows," was only apparent and often in full contrast with the outcome of the trials: Sentences were usually slow in coming and often practically nonexistent, a situation rarely found in the law courts of other cities. The prescribed fine of twenty-five gold "scudi," a sum that could hardly be counted on from the penniless purses of charlatans, was often considerably reduced, if not completely dodged, for a pardon could easily be obtained from the grand duke of Tuscany. An eighteenth-century document states, "All these penalties [are] for the most part unfeasible because the transgressors, who exercise the profession of medicasters, are usually poor and wretched, and also because the condemned further appeal for a pardon and obtain it."[27] For repeat offenders, the penalties were even more severe, such as exile or prison, but usually all was resolved with a few days in jail, a period that usually lasted only for the time of the trial.

The proceedings of one trial recount that "a young man of the apparent age of thirty, stout around the waist, of a stature more short than tall, dressed all in black with a Skirt to his Knee, is taken from prison" and brought before the reunited council and College of Physicians. When asked for his generalities, the young man states, "I am Florentine, and my profession now is to mount a bench." For a month he had been roaming around Siena and the nearby villages and countryside with a certain "Doctor" Lombardo, a fellow that he met in Leghorn. To avoid incrimination, he declares that he is a simple subordinate, hired because "I possess an easy chatter," an indispensable quality for a charlatan.

While the two were selling remedies in the square, they met a man "from the Customs, who asked for medical help for his poor wife." The following day the two charlatans arrived at his house and, after fully restoring themselves, examined the woman. Interrogating her at length about her disturbances, Doctor Lombardo promised to cure her in twenty days. The charlatan's physic consisted of an oil, to be drunk every morning in a cup of broth, mixed with a special liquid that he himself had prepared. But after this treatment, the wife showed no improvement; on the contrary, she "lost flesh," even though the charlatan had promised that she would become "as fat as himself."

The patient, who probably had malaria, confirmed that she had been bedridden for almost six years with a sickness that made her sweat. The judges seemed uncertain what to do. How could they condemn the charlatan if the disease were incurable, and even licensed physicians were unable to make the woman's health improve? As the trial dragged on, the customs officer seemed particularly anxious to be reimbursed for his expenses and sent a petition to the grand duke asking that he be at least given back his deposit. At last, the court condemned the "doctor" to the payment of a fine of "twenty-five of gold." At this point, the charlatan sent a heartfelt plea to the chief physician and the counselors, reminding them that because he was "so miserable and imprisoned, he is unable to pay the aforementioned fine," and begged them to give him "charity of this penalty."

The sentence arrived: The deposit would be given back to the customs officer and the charlatan would pay the sole expenses of the trial, but as a final gesture of good will, the College of Physicians decided that the "charlatan receive grace of the fourth pertaining to our faculty."[28]

A Plague-Spreader

Recurrences of plague were particularly difficult periods for charlatans. As soon as there was the merest hint of "corruption and infection of the air," they ran the risk of being suspected, arrested, and imprisoned. Every vagabond aroused the anxiety, the apprehension, the terror that he could carry with him the "sticky atoms of the plague." In the "Bans for Provisions in the Matter of Plague," published in November, 1629, and in July, 1673, Cardinal Pallavicino, "venerable legate of Bologna," decreed that "admission to Gypsies, Vagabonds, Rascals and Beggars" should be prevented. For "similar riffraff," the law, besides a fine, dispensed "three strappado and also Prison according to their quality: fifty straps for Putti [children], and lashes for Women." The same penalty was reserved for those who gave them lodgings, such as "Innkeepers, Publicans, Stablekeepers, and Hostelers."[29]

A poor merchant who came from afar could be transformed by the public imagination into a malicious plague spreader. Girolamo Giannelli probably never got over the terrible adventure that befell him in the city of Volterra on a warm day in August, 1630. At that time the humble charlatan wandered from village to village, selling pins, loose sheets printed with stories, and simple remedies such as "sealed earth" against fevers. More because of the terrible heat than out of devotion, he had the unfortunate idea of entering the cathedral and dipping his hands into the basin of holy water. This act was sufficient to arouse the suspicion of some onlookers; he was a stranger and therefore doubtlessly intended to contaminate the water with poisons and powders hidden amongst his wares. Immediately denounced to the bailiffs of the Bargello, Giannelli was arrested and thrown into prison. The acts of the interrogation before the Florentine commissioners describe "one of average stature, accused of having bewitched the Holy Water of the Cathedral and of other churches" — a serious accusation, for the scaffold awaited those who attempted to spread contagion. Under the pressing questions of the judges, the poor man defended himself as best he could, but the judges insisted that he was lying, for witnesses stated that he was seen skulking around a confessional for no apparent reason. He had to explain what he intended to do with all those "papers and things" that he carried on his person. The charlatan maintained that his "things" were roots of horst for toothache, oil of lavender, and "alum of scorched rock that he used for an eyewash, and sealed earth that was useful for fever."[30] His remedies were similar to those of Roberto Rosaccio, a physician well liked by the Medici court, and perhaps for this reason, poor Giannelli was at last released. It can be imagined that after this dangerous adventure, the poor quack preferred to return to his former trade of shoemaker.

CHAPTER 2

Grand Entertainments

On a beautiful spring day of the year 1778, the Council and Secret Authority of the Grand Duke of Tuscany granted a license to Giovanni Antonio Scolari, a charlatan from Bologna nicknamed "Gambacorta" (Shortleg), who was passing through Pistoia to "perform his art." It was the long-awaited permit to "sell balms and specifics and other medical commodities during the day" and to recite "comedies and jokes" with his company of players in the evening. But the permit contained a categorical warning: "The show must end when the musical opera at the Teatro dei Risvegliati of this city begins."[1]

From the latter part of the Middle Ages, the trade of medical charlatans was increasingly associated with the art of the comedian. Spectacles and farces in the open squares were an indispensable complement to their art, a clever artifice to attract crowds for the purpose of selling medicinal wares. For centuries, the shows put on by charlatans were oddly similar to popular theater: The charlatan and the actor led the same errant lives, and the professional success of each depended on his ability to prepare a captivating stage setting and recite in public; both used the same gestures, the same words, the same ploys, the same allusions, the same vulgar ambiguities.

An Englishman's Description of Quacks in Venice

A curious Englishman, Thomas Coryat, wrote a keen and lively description of Venetian charlatans at the beginning of the seventeenth century. After arranging the contents of a huge "trunke, which is replenished with a world of newfangled trumperies," the charlatans behave like a regular company of actors: The men mask themselves like "fooles in a play," and the numerous and fine-looking women dress themselves according to the part to which they have been assigned. At the end of a long vocal and instrumental introduction, the "Captaine and ring-leader" begins an interminable discourse, designed to exalt the virtues of his medical remedies, his drugs, and his beauty products: "The head Mountebanke at every time that he delivereth out any thing, maketh an extemporall speech, which he doth eftsoones intermingle with such savory jests (but spiced now and then with singular scurrility) that they minister passing mirth and laughter to the whole company, which perhaps may consist of a thousand people that flocke together about one of their stages." He tells of a "black gowned, blind Mountebanke, noted to be a singular fellow for singing extemporall songes, and for a pretty kind of musicke that he hath made with two bones betwixt his fingers."

Like every open-air merchant, after the give and take of bargaining, the quacks at last lower the price of their wares "from ten crowns to only four gazzettes." "These merry fellowes doe most commonly continue two good houres upon the stage and at last when they have fedde the audience with such passing variety of sport, that they have even cloyed with the superfluity of their conceits, and have sold as much ware as they can, they remove their trinkets and stage till the next meeting." Coryat, a disenchanted admirer, gave special attention to these spectacles, for he was a professional barker and therefore had good reason to study the quacks' techniques with particular application.[2]

In the seventeenth century, Italian charlatans gained such a reputation in England and France that these countries became a land of conquest for many intrepid healers: In Ben Jonson's famous comedy, Volpone impersonates an Italian quack, the Scoto Mantovano. The author may have been inspired by a real Italian quack, a certain Dionisio Scoto.

Returning to Venice after months of absence, the "Mantovano" finds his coveted place in front of the procurators' office in Saint Mark's square occupied by a rival. Without losing heart, he humbly retires to "an obscure nook of the square," declaring that it is much better there, for "far from the clamor of the 'canaglia,' it will be a scene of pleasure and delight." Only a tiny amount of his precious "Oyle of Scoto" is left, which alone has the virtue "to fortify the most indigest and crude stomach, ay blood, applying only a warm napkin to the place, after the unction and fricace...." It heals "the 'mal caduco,' cramps, convulsions, paralyses, epilepsy's, 'tremorcordia,' retired nerves, ill vapours of the spleen, stoppings of the liver, the stone, the strangury, 'hernia ventosa,' 'iliaca passio'"; and "easeth the torsion of the small guts, and cures melancholia hypocondriaca, being taken and applied according to my printed receipt." "O, Health! Health! the blessing of the rich/the riches of the poor/who can buy thee at too dear a rate, since there is no enjoying the world without thee? Be not so sparing of your purses, honorable gentlemen, as to abridge the natural course of life. For this is the physician, this the medicine; this counsels, this cures; this gives the direction, this works the effect."[3]

Other amusing examples of charlatanesque rhetoric can be found in satires written between the eighteenth and nineteenth centuries. Gioachino Belli wrote this parody of a famous charlatan haranguing the crowd: "Cultured and respectable Publick, sickly Publick of Rome, rejoice at last, for the celebrated, most humble Gambalunga is with you. Here is your Servant, that you have so long awaited, that braggart of Medicine, who with the Aid of heaven has performed innumerable operations for the profit of poor Humanity...." "Come now, oh Cancers; hurry Stones and Gravel; make yourselves known, oh occult Diseases ... for I, with the egregious virtue of my miserable ignorance, strengthened by the help of the Almighty, will know how to force you back inside, silencing any rival of my famous doctrine with the renown of my marvels.... I can nothing, I know nothing, I say nothing of myself, but allow them to speak, if they have breath, the Universities of Paris, the Colleges of London, the Gymnasiums of Lipsia, the Chairs of St. Petersburg, the Faculties of Berlin, the Surgeries of Turin, the Clinics of Munich, the Observatories of Dresden, the Hospitals of Madrid, the Cemeteries of Lisbon; speak out oh Laboratories of Stockholm, Workshops of Brussels, Streets of Copenhagen, Mosques of Constantinople, Cafes of Genoa, Canals of Venice, Squares of Milan, Docks of Naples, and the Grand Dukes' Square in Florence, and the Agonal Circus (Piazza Navona) and the Pantheon of this eternal city...."

He offers to "operate, I say, with impunity and with my eyes closed, on any human or inhuman body, Medicine, Surgery, Natomy, Pathology, Plebotomy [phlebotomy], Geography, Pharmacy, Orthography, Gastronomy ... Obstetrics, Veterinary, Botany, Mechanics, Hydraulics, and finally, natural and universal History."[4]

Rhetoric, Acrobats and Animal Trainers

The successful charlatan secured the most strategic and sought-after position in the squares of large cities and busy towns; often, his arrival was announced by the rolling of drums or a pandemonium of trumpets, violas and kettledrums. The acclaimed healer, accompanied by a follow-

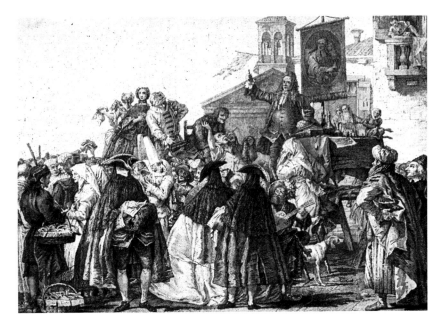

A festive air with masks and players around a charlatan's platform in Venice. G. Leonardis, from a drawing by G. Tiepolo (1765). U.S. National Library of Medicine, Bethesda, MD.

ing of servants in livery and barkers declaiming his excellence, descended from a sumptuously decorated carriage pulled by fancily caparisoned horses, their hooves painted with gold. The sale of remedies proceeded alongside the business of entertainment: Companies of actors and masks recited comedies and bawdy farces or sang or told lively stories for the amusement of the gathering. The musical accompaniment served to attract the crowd and sometimes was indispensable to cover the screams of the unfortunate victim subjected to a surgical operation or the extraction of a tooth.

Often a banner with the charlatan's insignia waved above the platform: Some exhibited paintings with various symbols taken from astrology, or motifs of birds, monsters, or fantastic animals. The more modern charlatans, in tune with the times, exhibited rough anatomical drawings, confirmation of their competence and scientific reliability; their entire therapeutic arsenal of ampoules, retorts, beakers, decanters and pots was displayed along with their surgical instruments.

The public stood entranced by comedies, singing, sharp exchanges and witty dialogues, or gaped with admiration at dancers, fencers, magicians, acrobats or skilled tightrope walkers. Anything strange, any natural curiosity could serve to attract their attention. A tarantula, a scorpion or some other rare creature like a regulus snake, with tiny ears and a squamous head the size of a melon, or a "deaf asp" or a crocodile brought from Egypt or an "Indian lizard" could be exhibited on the charlatan's platform. Expert taxidermists fashioned deadly beasts with consummate ability, terrifying monsters stuffed with straw.

In etchings and paintings, a petulant monkey is often portrayed beside the platform where the charlatan is performing. In medieval tradition this animal was used to represent imitation.[5] Saint Hildegard, the twelfth century Benedictine abbess whose "Physica" became a celebrated treatise on medicine, indicated the monkey, this strange creature who is neither entirely animal nor entirely human, as the most appropriate symbol of false medical knowledge.

Some charlatans were accomplished animal tamers; the Florentine archives mention a "Turk" who performed in the squares with a trained bear. An illustrious seventeenth-century naturalist refers, in "The Marvels of Nature," to a "circolatore" who performed with a dog which would pick up rings thrown on the ground by bystanders and return each to its owner. But the dog's specialty was to demonstrate "amongst women those who were married, those who were virgin and those who were widows, by touching their clothes."[6]

The philosopher Benedetto Croce remembered, during his own childhood, the exhibitions of mountebanks with their animals in the squares of Naples, those same spectacles that had been seen in the seventeenth century.[7]

Players

Numerous anecdotes of popular folklore recall a multitude of humble charlatans, disguised as extravagant and playful orators. These merchants of remedies could transform themselves at will into strolling players, clever at inventing exhilarating dialogues, parodies, or an infinite number of jokes. They appeared in the city squares, in out-of-the-way towns, in the countryside as plebeian actors or eccentric pranksters whose gags were peppered with coarse scurrility. So much effort, such tireless fantasy were necessary for these modest "makers of spectacles" just to be able to sell a few remedies at the end of the show. They had to surpass all other rivals in quick-wittedness, constantly inventing novelties and taking advantage of each situation with inexhaustible imagination.

They were so clever, so appealing that Garzoni had to reluctantly admit: "They have gained such credit with the vulgar mob that the crowds hasten to applaud them more than they do the excellent orators of the divine Word and the honored professors of the Sciences and the Arts." He describes "Fortunato" and his company "shooting out nonsense, and entertaining the rabble every evening from the twenty-second to the twenty-fourth hour of the day [three to five p.m.], inventing tales, dreaming up stories … arguing amongst themselves, then making peace and singing." On the other side of the square is "Burattino" (Puppet), with a strong Bolognese accent, dressed "in a porter's sack, a little cap on his head that makes him look like an imp." The crowd pushes; common folk and gentlemen laugh until they nearly burst at his ridiculous, rambling speech, at his hilarious wisecracks cried out in dialect, "with that monkey's voice." He makes a caricature of an erudite doctor, "reciting all his doctoral privileges out of place, pretending to be a Chief Physician without science…." The "Tuscan," with a girl, parades along an improvised ramp, talking on and on in "Florentine tongue" and making sleights of hand, while "The Milanese," dressed like a noble gentleman, velvet cap with a white plume "like a Guelf," pretends to be in love with his servant. "This one (the servant) instead makes vulgar gestures in his face," but when he sees his master's rivals "he becomes all paralytic, and shaking with fear, soils himself on the stage," then runs away leaving the Milanese all flustered in the middle of the gathering with his "vials and boxes full of his medical remedies." There is "Master Lione," "graduated," and the "Blind Man" from Forlì, and Zen from the Vineyard, who makes sleights and "motions with his body"; more gibberish follows as "the nobility laughs, the common folk guffaw, the bumpkins nearly die." There is even a Turk, an acrobat and expert trainer, a personage who would have appealed to Fellini, who makes his little dog sing: "ut, re, mi, sol, fa…."[8]

These ragged jesters, who lived by selling their medicinal wares, knew how to interpret the feelings and needs of the rabble: Their pranks, their caricatures and buffoonery were meant to provoke good humor, to release merriment. They used laughter as the most effective propitiatory means against sickness, anxiety, and misery.

Pomp, music and ladies

In addition to the lower orders of quacks, the solitary artists and jesters, the ridiculous and vulgar buffoons that Garzoni so accurately described, there were brilliant and more fortunate charlatans, genuine leading actors. Ever more frequently the urban public could attend grandiose spectacles put on by companies of seasoned players. The magnificence of the scenery and costumes made these recitals even more seductive; this time the fun did not depend on one actor alone but was assured by a generous cast of comedians, jesters, singers, dancers, jugglers, and pretty ladies.

The charlatans of higher rank enjoyed the protection of the royalty, the clergy, the magistrates, the affluent and the nobility, who retained the most strategic corners of the city for their performances. Some entertainments were reserved, as when the comedy was presented in "the private palace of a Gentleman."

The head charlatan was no longer alone in front of his audience, but performed with his company; during the intermissions, elixirs, juleps, herbal mixtures and electuraies, whose princely cost matched the splendor of the spectators' names and the elegance of the show, were offered to the audience. The charlatan, now transformed into the leading comedian, elegantly dressed in an ornate and lavish costume resplendent with gold necklaces, sword at his side, directed his company with the talent of a real actor. The platform became the grand stage where the comedy unfolded, where he could "hugely amuse the assembly, now with cutting wit, now with marvelous imitations, now with extravagant inventions, now with other simple means to cause relish."

In these companies, the presence of one or more ladies was fundamental for the felicitous outcome of the show: The minds of the spectators were enticed, and their enjoyment increased. Charlatans understood that "without Women they will be thought to offer nothing and to be judged Comedians worthy of little applause…." Expert players, they knew by experience that "a woman seen and heard gives pleasure with her singing and playing, and most of the time restores the audience with various marvelous movements of her body." When she asks graciously for a reward, the spectators do not "hesitate to give it to her readily."

A racy chronicle in the Florentine archives, dated during the year 1616, tells of a certain "Vettoria," whose salary of fifteen scudi a month was paid for by a company of charlatans: She "sings and dances and leaps" and was such a dazzling actress that she had to be accompanied home by four bouncers so as not to be squeezed in the crush of admirers, a sign of enormous celebrity, just like any modern diva.

Vettoria was a "courteous lady, dressed like a boy, clean and neat," who attracted a huge crowd with "somersaults … with divine dancing, with singing so soothing, and a glance so beautiful that in its sweetness [it] moves everyone to compassion, and being all put into a slumber, they cry out sighing … oimeè, oimeeè my heart, what is this? Especially old men, who look on her with their mouths open, because they would like to play games with her and give her a licking."⁹

During the Counter-Reformation, the presence of women caused scandal and protests from the ecclesiastical authorities, so that even some powerful sovereigns were reluctant to grant permits for those comedies in which females participated. The grand duke of Tuscany, Ferdinand II, received many petitions from charlatans who meekly pleaded for licenses to organize companies employing extras of both sexes, but he seemed doubtful about creating other problems for himself with the clergy and above all with Maffeo Barberini, the austere Pope Urban VIII. In 1627, Francesco Scarione, a Bolognese charlatan, requested a permit to "mount the stage with masked and unmasked personages, with music on workdays as well as holidays." The reason for this magnificent show was to sell "oil for cold pains, compresses for the stomach, ointments to increase milk, rinses for the mouth and external things." The grand duke granted the authorization, but beneath his signature, a large "F," an unequivocal warning is written: "granted without women."¹⁰

A thick crowd of idlers watched the shows that took place in the squares without paying; they went to see the charlatans as they would have attended the theater. "Thus goes the world," acknowledged the Jesuit priest Giovanni Domenico Ottonelli: "[A] company of these [charlatans] sometimes appear[s] in a City and spread[s] the word that they want to serve the public, selling excellent secrets and reciting beautiful Comedies, and this to provide amusement and pleasure without payment." For a more select public, who paid for a ticket, the recital often took place indoors in a large room or hall, where there were "benches, or stools, or chairs where one could hear more comfortably." This dogged censor of morals attended a huge number of comedies presented by players of every type, even though he refused to condone these exhibitions, which he judged dangerously immoral, contrivances and reflections of Satan. In his ponderous work "Of Christian Moderation in the Theater," he harshly admonishes those "modern and immoderate charlatans" who use "obscenities of gesture and speech" in order to make an amusing spectacle.¹¹

Despite his exaggerated rigor, Ottonelli provides an invaluable description of how these elaborate entertainments were performed. "At a convenient hour" of each day, the charlatanesque spectacle begins; first the buffoon appears, playing and singing to lure the public, then other funny players join him, with ladies, and all together they perform "a mixture of popular attractions." When the show is well under way, the archcharlatan appears; his task is to recite the miracles of his secret remedies. If the sale goes well, a "Lady offers her confections, or some other kindness" as thanks to the public. Then, the main part begins: "a dramatic recitation or comedy which entertains the people for the space of two hours, with gaiety, with laughter, with amusement." Ottonelli almost always finds occasion for sin in the comedies that employ many ladies. He admits that it is not the fault of the charlatans alone, but of the lewd spectators as well, who begin to get restless at the start of the show and shout in a ribald way, demanding to see the buffoon and especially the "Maidservant," yelling for the foul language to begin: the same coarse uproar that preceded the pelvic roll of the "chanteuse" in popular curtain risers of a more recent era.

Ottonelli relates the scandalous episode of a "virtuous Gentlewoman" who "found so many thorns amongst comic flowers, and heard, and saw such numerous, indecent obscenities, that she blushed for shame more than once." According to the implacable moralist, these "Comedians" are in effect almost always "indecent"; the charlatans "offend God with impure fingerings, and with dishonest words." He recalls a young man who "stated with the utmost conviction that he had committed about ten thousand sins for having gone eight or ten times to the platform in the square where the Charlatans with their Women performed these same, obscene representations." The appearance of women who speak of love on the public stage is "an obscene, scandalous and dangerous medium for the many who are weak in spirit." "A wise man," in the end declared, "hearing constantly flesh, flesh, flesh, a man would have to be made of iron." Ottonelli approves of Monsignor Saladino, the bishop of Syracuse, who forbad an impudent charlatan, peddler of secrets, to hold his spectacle in the square with "Women of the usual scandalous qualities." When the arrogant quack replied that he would not obey the order because he had many "very ample permits granted by Supreme Lords" in his possession, the bishop threatened to have him "publickly whipped, for no Lord is so great that he can give authorization to lead the lambs of his flock into sin."[12]

Rivalry in the Squares between Charlatans and Clergy

In the seventeenth century, it was often risky for actors to perform in recitals that contained obscenity. The companies that played in Naples ordered any actor who heard an oath from the mouth of a colleague to denounce him without delay. Every player had the obligation to confess himself at least once a year.

Disputes and rivalry were rife between charlatans and clergy eager to prevail in the squares: The "art of speaking" was as indispensable for the clergyman, who preached from his pulpit, as it was for the charlatan, who declaimed from his platform. Charlatans often disturbed the reunions of preachers with their shouting. Benedetto Croce told of a Protestant bishop, a certain Burnet, who, arriving in Naples, saw a Jesuit in the square "call the people to himself and lead them in procession, until, arriving at a place where a charlatan was selling his remedies, he climbed upon a platform and started entertaining the audience with jokes."[13]

Many ecclesiastics in Naples did not approve of the profane shows that were put on in the busy squares. A preacher, deserted by his listeners for a charlatan who was playing Pulcinella, called them all back, waving his crucifix and exclaiming: "Here, here, for this is the true Pulcinella!" Clashes often occurred because the clergy, by ancient tradition and in spite of an interdiction by the ecclesiastical authorities, often practiced every type of cure below board and administered various remedies, exacting payment without qualms.

Charlatans not only had to deal with the protests of physicians and chemists and the competition of friars, they also faced the wrath of authors and actors of comedies. Perrucci, author of a book on theatrical art, rose in defense of the latter, adding his own voice to their indignation by railing against those extemporaneous players who perform "improvised comedies in the public squares, mangling the subjects, speaking out of turn, gesticulating like lunatics, and even worse, mouthing a thousand obscenities and oaths, all to extract a sordid gain ... selling fake cooked oils, antidotes that poison, and remedies that make nonexistent ills appear."

Some charlatans organized shows with jugglers "inside a mock canvas castle" or a puppet theater in which there were "small figures that are made to gesture and say words with much effectiveness to excite pleasure and laughter in the Spectators." Ottonelli admits that this amusement, when performed without obscenity, "remains within the terms of a curious and pleasurable popular entertainment," but when "one hears ugly words, or one sees dishonest deeds, then the Puppets in the castle serve the Devil in Hell to ruin many Souls ... and the Juggler, and the Charlatan is an ignominious, and infamous Minister of Dishonesty, and Go-Between for eternal damnation."

Other charlatans measured themselves with "Marvelous Amusements," with sleights of hand or feats such as "walking, or dancing upon a cable, imitating the strength of Hercules, doing somersaults, flying from one place to another with a rope ... walking with hands and feet in the air, making a beast dance or jump, or showing a woman dressed like a man: deceiving the eyes with tricks like lifting a huge weight with their hair, or wounding some part of the body and then quickly becoming healed." Ottonelli remembers a "riskful Turk," a funambulist who let someone "beat on his chest with a hammer, as if on a hard anvil." And then, with the sole strength of his shoulders, pulled a "huge pole out of the ground." By doing this, he earns "good money to take to the Mecca."[14] Any form of spectacle, any exhibition, any sort of dexterity of mind or body could aid the charlatan; amazed spectators watched the vaulting funambulists, transfixed, even if they seemed demons rather than men.[15]

The gravest suspicion of immorality fell on "the Ridiculous Charlatan, the Satirical, the Facetious, the Comical, and the Obscene." The first of these "laughs at his fellows for their defects"; some are coprophagists, who have no compunctions about swallowing, or making someone else swallow, excrement. The audience's guffaws are the reward for these trivial pranks, which make even those who have been duped laugh. Another type of charlatan makes "silly tomfoolery, ingenious and cheerful bagatelles"; this buffoon recites "mere and foolish jokes." All are in danger of sin, but there is no doubt in Ottonelli's mind that Hell's worst punishments are reserved for the "obscene" charlatan.[16]

Ottonelli did not always agree with Scipione Mercuri; on occasion, he even considered his own opinions too rigorous. Ottonelli believed that condemnation was justifiable only if the theatrical charlatans went against Christian virtues; Mercuri's disapproval of charlatans was systematically without appeal and regarded every action that the "libelers, gasbags, whorers, gamblers" performed.

How can one entrust one's health, Mercuri insisted, to someone who practices medicine with buffoons or uses a spectacle of puppets, or still worse, is accompanied by prostitutes? "Oh poor Vulgar folk," he dramatically exclaims, "Medicine is virtue; therefore to sell it along with comedy is to butcher it." The charlatans' incapacity and ignorance are so great that "the patient either dies, or remains an invalid; if any remedy of theirs ever helped one, it harmed a thousand." The physician's indignation was probably due in part to a financial reasoning; Mercuri was not insensible to money and had only words of contempt for patients who did not pay their bills, or even worse, tried to cheat the doctor with a "shaved" coin, a coin in which some of the silver had been filed off; these patients were "a throng of dreamers, who think that they can save money by consulting charlatans, and instead forfeit both their purses and their lives."[17]

Ottonelli's judgment was more even tempered. He believed that in the midst of those "undisciplined, dissolute, ignorant thieves of other peoples' money" there could even be some "Gentlemen," who possess "true and experimented secrets" that have been tried in different places, often with success. Perhaps he had once fallen ill and, disappointed by the therapeutical impotence of his doctors, had tried some charlatan's remedy with satisfaction, enough to recognize that it is false "to say that whoever buys medical remedies from any Charlatan commits an error." There are some charlatans who are "very virtuous, and give pleasure with the Art, and help with the sale of good remedies." Ottonelli was convinced that many of their remedies "are efficacious, and good for some infirmities."[18]

Poisonous Asps and the "People of Saint Paul"

The inevitable brawls amongst charlatans, their contentions and rivalries, their craving to cause excitement and stir up passions in the onlookers sometimes resulted in cruel exhibitions of "blood and fire." Some of the more reckless quacks did not hesitate to inflict wounds on themselves: cuts, bleeding sores or burns caused by boiling pitch, which they promptly healed with their secret unguents, all in plain view of the crowd. Clever illusionists, rather than plain foolhardy, they made what seemed like serious injuries disappear by using their miraculous balms, or they mysteriously avoided death after swallowing potent poisons or being bitten by venomous snakes.

Dangerous experiments with snakes were among the most common exhibitions that could be seen in the city and village squares. Nothing could cause more excitement or wonder than a charlatan who fearlessly proffered some part of his body to a poisonous reptile's bite. From the time of Galen, charlatans had let themselves be bitten by snakes in order to prove that they possessed infallible remedies against venom. Mercuri explained the procedure: "Before handling the serpents, they grease their hands with an ointment made of juice of tarragon, juice of asphodel roots, leaves of broadbeans, juniper berries, hare's brain, oil from the seeds of wild horseradish." The poisonous snakes remain "dazed by their virtues and cannot bite." Charlatans often captured asps and vipers in the dead of winter, when they are less likely to attack; they also used another ruse, goading "the snakes to bite a piece of meat … until they lose their natural poison."[19]

Piero Andrea Mattioli, the Sienese physician, explained that charlatans "spit on their [the serpents'] heads after fasting, which humiliates them more than a little, for the saliva of man is naturally contrary to their poisonous nature." The learned doctor had to reluctantly admit that sometimes, "for a certain virtue of Heaven, acquired by some influx of the fixed stars," the execrable quacks do not get bitten, and if they are, the bite is often harmless.[20] The truth was actually much simpler: All they had to do was remove the vipers' fangs or extract the venom glands and then take care that the trick was not discovered.

Platforms, stages, shacks and puppet theaters were concentrated in the wide square in front of the Angiovin Castle in Naples, a favorite gathering place for ciaravoli or ciaraldi, who congregated "with a box full of snakes, showing them off and playing with them, and selling poultices." Charlatans who acquired great familiarity with reptiles became snake tamers; a certain Maestro Moretto imprudently kept many serpents in his house, "neither more nor less than good fathers do with their family"; but one day his body was discovered "extinguished by bites."

In 1610, a Florentine charlatan was advertising the merits of a remedy that he hoped to sell to the public: He picked up a "very wild viper" and let it bite a part of his chest very near his heart." Everyone expected the antidote to protect him from the viper's venom, but the charlatan was so busy haranguing the audience that he forgot to take his remedy. The crowd began to murmur, "either he will die, or else the viper has no venom, in which case the charlatan is a wily trickster.... [T]hen the People started to rant against him, and scream and insult him and almost made him come down off the stage by throwing rocks. The wretch made off confused, and found disgrace, which was well deserved for his deceiving insolence and presumption."

When charlatans challenged each other in the squares, it was not always a simulated exhibition created solely to impress the public. If the two rivals exchanged their poisonous snakes, there was always the chance that one of them could really be poisoned, although this rarely happened, for it was generally the rule that secret agreements had been made beforehand.

Some wandering quacks claimed to be descendants of the Marsi, an ancient Italian people who had been taught how to make themselves immune to the poisonous bites of reptiles by the son of Medea. They wore the image of a snake impressed on their flesh and maintained that they could heal the unfortunate victims of venomous bites by touch alone. Some charlatans called themselves "People of Saint Paul," profiting from an early Christian legend of a miracle that the saint was believed to have performed on the island of Malta.

"I have observed marveilous strange matters done by some of these Mountebanks," Thomas Coryat remembers, "[f]or I saw one of them holde a viper in his hand, and play with his sting a quarter of an hour together, and yet receive no hurt; though another man should have beene presently stung to death with it. He made us all believe that the same viper was lineally descended from the generation of that viper that lept out of the fire upon S. Paul's hand, in the Island of Melita now called Malta and did him no hurt; and told us moreover that it would sting some, and not others."[21] There was a common belief that members of some families possessed the ability to render poisonous snake bites harmless: The so-called snake handlers and the Saint Dominicans, named for Saint Dominique of Sora, who shared this power with Saint Paul, were amongst the chosen.

"Some of these vagabonds," noted Moryson, "carry serpents with them and sell remedies against their bites, that they call grace of Saint Paul, who remained immune to the viper's bite."[22] The physician Mattioli wrote, "The same fraud has then remained to quacks of our times who call themselves (and they lie through their teeth) of the house of Saint Paul. They swear that they are able to heal by solely touching the unfortunate wretch who has been bitten by serpents."

Scipione Mercuri scoffs at those impostors who claim to be descendants of Saint Paul: "[Y]et even a worm in the form of man, a vile buffoon, a charlatan, claims to be his relative...."

Ancient and Modern Shows with Snakes

The painting on a fifteenth-century marriage chest, preserved in the museum of the Bargello, depicts the "Procession of the Banners," held in Florence on the feast day of Saint John, patron saint of the city: An elegant, opulent parade, in which a group of gentlemen are riding on white steeds, proceeds through the square in front of the cathedral. On the left-hand side of the square, in front of the baptistry named for the "Beautiful Saint John," the figure of a charlatan can be seen, upright upon his stand. He is an impressive man with a long beard, dressed in red like a physician, his waist tied with a wide sash from which a purse hangs. The artist has drawn him in the act of declaiming the virtues of his remedies to the crowd; in his right hand he tightly clasps a long black snake that writhes in wide coils. In the other hand he holds up a small box with his precious arcanum. A large group of Florentines, elegantly dressed for the occasion, seem curious, intrigued more by the charlatan than by the splendid ceremony that is unfolding on the other side of the square.

Five centuries later, in the spring of 1922, a scene akin to the one depicted on the ancient chest took place a hundred yards or so from the Baptistry, in front of the severe, unfinished facade of the basilica of San Lorenzo; a charlatan in flesh and blood, surrounded by a crowd of commoners, was noticed by professor Andrea Corsini, a Florentine doctor and writer, who described him in his book on medical quacks: "He was a huge man, standing erect on a stool in front of a table covered by a long carpet on which a suitcase was placed. His head was uncovered, a little bald in the front, but with a long mane of black curly hair that swayed violently, following the vehemence of his gestures and of his speech, a shock of hair that reminded me of certain African tribes that I had seen in Morocco. When I arrived, he had taken a long blackish snake out of the suitcase and clasped it near the head with the fingers of his left hand. It writhed, trying to escape and to bite, and he, as he spoke, brought the index finger of his right hand close, towards which it lunged; sometimes he allowed himself to be bitten, and when the snake was well attached, he would leave it hanging from his finger until, with his free hand he would pry its mouth open and go back to grasping it by the neck as before. Then he would clean his finger on a towel, as if drying off blood, which I however was unable to see: probably the animal had been deprived of its teeth."

"In the meantime he kept repeating that if anyone present had allowed himself to be bitten by a similar animal he soon would have 'returned his soul to God and his body to the earth.' Then he went on to say that he had not come to ask for money, or to sell anything, but only to propagandize, to make known, how necessary it is to take care of one's person and especially one's mouth. As he said this, he bent over to draw a package out from under the table; this he opened, along with a small box contained inside; from this he took a small amount of powder which he put in a glass, and poured pure water over it, very pure, with no deceit, and shook the mixture. Then he made a thousand faces to show how his mouth felt fresh, perfumed, and how his teeth had become full of force and vigor."[23] Corsini, along with the others in the crowd, purchased this prodigious powder, a mixture that turned out to be talcum and kaolin. It was a pardonable fraud: After all, the charlatan had only advertised dental hygiene.

Trials by Blood and Fire

Since the crowds were increasingly attracted by the charlatan' perilous exhibitions, a request was made in one of the petitions addressed to the Venetian superintendents of health in June of 1693 to forbid these cruel demonstrations: "Perceiving the most Illustrious and Most Excellent Chief Superintendent and Superintendents of Health how these experiences, that by Mountebanks, Charlatans, and other persons are practiced in the Squares with scandal of the righteous, are against Christian and public charity." The broadsheet calls attention to the imprudent and dangerous acts that were performed by the charlatans to attract and excite the crowds: "some making themselves brave to make cuts on their persons, receive considerable burns with oils, pitch, tar, and similar materials." The general chief physician of Milan, Giovanni Honorato Castiglione, forbad charlatans, in an ordinance dated January, 1676, "either to cut, or burn themselves, or allow themselves to be bitten by vipers on any part of the body, so that from such experiences the common folk be even more deceived."[24]

The rigorous prohibitions imposed on charlatans by the authorities were not necessarily a charitable act toward either the quacks or the common folk; they served, if at all, to prevent the public, thrilled by the remarkable shows, from rushing to buy the charlatans' remedies. Rather than an attempt to eliminate fraud, it was an endeavor to protect the purses of physicians and apothecaries.

Halfway through the seventeenth century, a celebrated Italian charlatan, Francesco Geronimo, accompanied by the "beautiful Galinette," performed at the palace court in Paris with extraordinary success. He called himself "Orvietano," a name that he shared with the potent, secret remedy that he sold. Soon the renown of his spectacular attractions caused the indignant suspicion of the physician Simon Sonnet De Courval, who wrote that with his own eyes he had seen the famous "Signore Hyeronimo," superbly attired, performing in the square with all his company, "whilst he showed off with a thousand lies and vain ostentation the occult virtues and admirable properties of his unguents, extracts, quintessences, distillations, calcifications, and other fantastic confections. "At the culmination of the spectacle, "to experiment the divine and admirable virtues of an unguent for burns," he placed a flaming torch on his hands until they were covered with horrible blisters. Then he applied his miraculous salve, and the blisters were healed as if by enchantment after two hours. De Courval contends that the quack had obviously used an "artificial" water that prevented the flame from burning his skin, even though it produced painless pustules that mysteriously disappeared "in dust and smoke," leaving the skin smooth and whole.

This was not the only astounding, self-inflicted ordeal; the charlatan wounded himself in the epigastrium with a sword, but the wound healed immediately after the application of his wondrous salve; this trick earned him immense fame and incredible success with his sales. De Courval, who had taken note of all his wounds, claimed that although they appeared healed, they were still fresh underneath, and it was only an act "to fool the world" and to collect money.[25]

As late as the end of the eighteenth century, an announcement in the *Gazzetta Toscana* advertised the hazardous exhibitions in Florence of Alessandro Granati: "He pulls teeth in the Square of the Grand Duke, with eyes blindfolded and sitting on a horse, he applies certain of his Balms that have a singular effect on all types of ailments. He proves this on his own body by cutting, piercing, burning his flesh, which heals with simple salves in less than twenty-four hours."

The need to amaze, to astound the public was so overwhelming that many charlatans inflicted real lesions on themselves: a grievous price to pay in order to triumph over other quacks for the favor of the public. "These may have been improper deceptions," wrote Piero Camporesi, "but the wounds that they inflicted on themselves were real. Pain and gore in order to sell just a few more jars of balm!"[26]

CHAPTER 3

"Wise is the peasant ... who does not go seeking a doctor's cure..."

Country Quacks versus Orthodox Physicians

For the masses of peasants who toiled in the fields, life was not the idyllic existence usually described in tales of Arcadia. Tormented by bullying masters and by incursions of disbanded soldiers and brigands, the peasants faced their greatest threat in the form of an infinite number of physical tribulations, diseases caused by the miserable standard of their lives, by malnutrition and filth. Historians speak vaguely of "fevers," which include "the quartan fever of ill fate," and catarrhs, complaints of the chest, infections from wounds, sore throat, pleurisy. The worthlessness of the cures proposed by official medicine, compounded with their inaccessible cost, forced these peasants to survive as best they could, accepting their lives with resignation. This is how a poet, Ercole Benitivoglio, saw their plight:

> But wise is the peasant, say I, who
> does not go seeking a doctor's cure...
> but leaves nature to resolve its course...
> For if Heaven has decided that thou shalt die,
> diet or lengthy cure will not make thee well.[1]

In addition to a multitude of dangerous scourges, there were minor, everyday plagues: scabies, a "very pertinacious and very painful mange," which caused scratching and impetigo and could become a serious problem. Many medical texts describe how diffused this aliment was throughout the poorer classes, a continual torment that was thought to be caused, according to the theories of the time, by "blood corrupted by internal vice of the humors." The real culprit was a loathsome mite that dug minuscule tunnels under the skin, a tiny worm that the "mangy" slaves in Leghorn dug out of each others' blisters with a needle. The medicine of humors had not discovered any effective remedy and prescribed the usual purgatives. Massages with mercury, an ancient empirical remedy, alternated with sulfur baths, gave the only temporary relief from the excruciating infestation.

Many physicians agreed that prescriptions for peasants should be different from those prescribed for city dwellers. "Warm urine of a virgin male-child," according to Marsilio Ficino, was an excellent remedy for fevers, though valid only for rustic clodhoppers; if they were unable to procure it, they could drink the urine of barnyard animals. Consensus justified the diversity of treatment for country folk: Just as the nobleman was handsome, the peasant was ugly and deformed. A caustic Thomaso Garzoni refers to "peasants sly as foxes, malicious as evil, damnable as devils." The peasant possesses neither "conscience nor reason, being an ox in his speech, an ass in his judgment, a nag in the intellect. He is rightfully baptized by all with such names as rustic, serf, snake in the grass, stupid yokel, worm, fleeced bumpkin, ignorant hick..."[2]

Poverty increased ignorance, and this in turn aggravated the darkest indigence; as time went by, the division between peasant and city dweller became progressively more pronounced. Professor Antonio Bertini, a conscientious seventeenth-century advocate of orthodox medicine, recounts an enlightening episode: The inhabitants of a rural area around a fortified castle belonging to the monks of St. Paul Beyond the Walls in Rome discovered, on consulting their death records, that there had been twice as many deaths amongst them since a salaried doctor had been appointed to their care. They sent a plea to Pope Innocent XI, begging him to send the doctor away. The pope, quite justifiably worried, considered the request reasonable. Professor Bertini defends the physician, whom he considers more naive than ignorant, for believing that "rough people, of a robust nature and of ruddy complexion," accustomed to fatigue and discomfort, are better able to stand continuous bleedings and tolerate any sort of medicine. Oddly, the opposite is true: "[B]ecause of their labors, peasants cannot accumulate a great fullness of blood" and suffer from bloodlettings more than city dwellers.[3]

The Idiotic Sawyer's Worm Grass

Although publicity in favor of well-known charlatans was tolerated to such an extent that the *Gazzetta Toscana* printed their advertisements without any verification, the police of the Tuscan grand duchy gave no respite to humble wandering quacks and lowly country medicasters. The charges that put the poor devils behind bars, more than to the zeal of the police were due to public or secret accusations made by envious local doctors who objected to being outdone by ignorant healers. The Florentine judiciary records, during the years of the grand duchy, contain indictments against simple medicasters who practiced in the countryside near the capital city. The accounts of the proceedings shed light on the way Florentine justice operated against a medical practice that was considered illegal and worthy of condemnation.

July 8, 1784, was an unlucky day for Lorenzo Bianchini, an elderly sawyer. Arrested in the early morning by the bailiffs of the College of Physicians, he was taken to the prisons of the supreme judiciary court of Florence. The accusations were serious: "[T]he said Lorenzo Bianchini of the commonality of S. Maria a Soffiano deceives simple and idiotic people with superstitions and impostures." One of the witnesses for the prosecution was the mayor; without mincing his words, he accused the old man of doctoring little children with secret remedies and superstitious divination, exacting from the ignorant country folk "at least a good lunch and some coins." The second witness, a police inspector, showed the court some irrefutable exhibits found in the defendant's pockets at the time of his arrest: dried herbs and a box of grease. The local doctor took the stand and accused the sawyer of practicing witchcraft; he was so incensed that he ridiculed the ignorance and credulity of the common people.

The following day, the defendant was brought in: "[a] man of regular height, thin of face, dressed in the usage of the country." The judges wanted to first investigate some facts, which if proven, could undoubtedly worsen the defendant's position. First he was asked the reason that he medicated these persons. The old man, careful not to fall into a trap, answered: "In truth, I did all for charity ... not for payment, and I always said, 'God give you merit.' That which I received was a piece of bread, a glass of wine from some, from others seven or eight cloves of garlic and onions, or a handful of beans. One gave me a coin to buy some tobacco." When interrogated as to whether he had ever tried to cure other sicknesses besides worms, he answered that he only tried to heal "some child beset by pain or other troubles." Other witnesses were brought in: One declared the old man to be honest, though "he is a vagrant, who insinuates himself into the homes of first one and then another where he finds some sick child, making the mother believe that it is bewitched." This testimonial was potentially dangerous: A suspicion could insinuate itself into the minds of the judges that the old man was not a poor, empirical herbalist but a country sorcerer, one of those magicians who recited litanies, made signs of the cross and "markings," and promised to remove the evil eye or chase out the devil, thus invading a field reserved for ecclesiastical exorcists. An animal trader's testimony was in the sawyer's favor: He was convinced that he was a courteous man and a good healer.

The trial drew to a close. The registrar's final relation was not altogether hostile toward the charlatan: an affair, he declared, about an "idiotic sawyer," reduced to poverty, who earned his bread thanks to the "excessive credulity of other idiots." With a formal order, the court magistrate instructed Bianchini "not to attempt to heal for the future.... [His] penalty [would be] a year of prison for transgression."[4]

The old man got off easily: He eluded the two charges that could have cost him dearly — exercising witchcraft and exchanging his services for money rather than out of charity for the poor. Once he had recovered from his fright, there is little doubt that the sawyer continued to go about until the end of his days successfully healing many "credulous idiots" that resorted to his cures.

Verminous Aggression

A multitude of afflictions were attributed to verminous aggression caused by worms supposedly generated by putrid or "pituitous" material. It was believed that worms lay sleeping quietly in the "verminous wheel," located in a corner of the intestine; if brusquely awoken, especially by a sudden fright, they came out of their refuge, causing confusion in the head and irritation in the guts. Unequivocal symptoms were a feverish shine in the eyes, screeching of the teeth, copious salivation, nausea and vomiting, and "wormy" breath, an ailment that nowadays would be attributed to acetonemia. Organic "consumption" was accompanied by a series of psychic troubles: swooning, vertigo, delirium, convulsions, epileptic attacks; these coincided, according to an ancient magical-religious theory, with the entrance of malignant spirits into the body of the possessed. "Sickness of the moon" occurs when children tremble and faint because a two-headed worm goes straight to their heart, "making them shake and many times killing them," wrote Don Alessio Piemontese in his "Secrets."[5] The demoniacal worms could enter or exit any part of the body along with the most unexpected and nauseous material: This information was not only a part of popular legend but can be found in learned medical treatises of the time.

As protection against verminous aggression, people had more faith in witches' charms, sorceresses' markings or charlatans' remedies than in physicians' dubious attempts to expel the worms with emetics from above or drastic enemas from below. It was arduous for the erudite doctors to try and conceal their ignorance: In the seventeenth century, a noble professor, Giovanni De Colli, lecturer at the celebrated University of Padua and chief physician to the Duke of Urbino, upheld the theory that "the Demons enter through the face, through food, through touch, with the breath, with vapor, fumes of poisonous aura, animal spirit." In general these are transmitted by "lamiae, lampuse, strigiae," monstrous women, allies of the devil, who arouse the worms with incantations or by putting strange images in the bed or in the clothing, or by making signs and enchantments. By means of their occult force, they provoke a malignant "consumption" in children and adults, "disturbing the body during sleep, changing the senses, exiting them to hatred, to love, to fury." The afflicted persons howl, "canes imitare latratu," or forget to speak their own dialect, talking instead in unknown and incomprehensible tongues. As a cure for the demoniacal bewitchment of children, the learned doctor prescribes prayer, holy water, saints' relics, or more down-to-earth inhalations made from stinking plants like rue or asphodel, which were believed to chase away demons. He suggests attaching to the crib "tintinnabula" or "crepunduia," the little bells made from gold, silver or coral in the shape of the wet nurse's nipples, that are shaken in front of a newborn baby. If the witchery does not retreat, the head of a black horse must be placed in a cubicle, and the skin of an eagle, a wolf, a lamb, or a sea lion wrapped around the body of the patient to extract the "maleficas causas." For those children fortunate enough to have been born to wealthy parents, he proposes another therapy, consisting in a "jeweled syrup" made from powdered precious stones; this probably had the immediate effect of rapidly delivering the child into the arms of the heavenly angels.[6]

At the end of the eighteenth century, Auguste Belloste, renowned physician and chief surgeon to Her Royal Majesty of Savoy, on observing "signs of worms" in the eyes of a patient, prescribed mercury pills dissolved in wine; after a short time, the woman vomited a "worm as long as a finger with a large head indeed." An annoyed Belloste recounts that unfortunately "the worm was thrown in the rubbish by the servants."[7] Another half-century was to elapse before hysteria would be recognized by official medicine.

Hipericum millefoliatum, or yarrow, was a small plant that, like St. John's wort, was believed to possess the power to destroy worms; its popular name was "demon-chaser"; these natural empirical herbs, which the old sawyer went seeking in the woods, were without a doubt a superior remedy against "verminous aggression."

The Charitable Miller's Mush

On October 2, 1784, the "Most Honorable Provider" of the quarter of Santa Maria Novella in Florence received judiciary proceedings against a miller from Lastra a Signa near Florence, a charlatan who was well known for his practice of illegal medicine. With equal tenacity, the same inspector who had accused the old sawyer delivered the indictment. But this time all the witnesses, in a unanimous chorus, declared that the defendant was not a dishonest cheat, eager for profit, but a veritable benefactor of the people. One witness told how the sick traveled to see the miller, even from far away, for, "being exceedingly stout (he) does not ordinarily go to homes to medicate, for he can barely move." His therapy consisted of mushes made of milk and bread or of simple herbs: With these remedies he healed patients that authorized doctors had been unable to help. The witnesses confirmed that the miller not only "never expects anything from any patient" but "treats all for charity" and even restores the most destitute with "mushes for alms and a little bread and a little wine ... and if someone brings him fruit, he gives it to them to refresh themselves, and thus pays for what was given." All his life the miller had "reasoned about different ailments and the virtues of herbs," with so much ability that "it is not possible either to name or to number" those whom he had benefited. "No one can recall any [amongst his patients], who died or complained of being badly treated." The enthusiastic popular testimonials disagreed however with the evidence brought by the local physician, who recounted that the miller had been curing people illegally for twenty-five years, exacting payment for his services and receiving gifts; many of his patients had been treated badly, and some had even died after his cures.

The beneficial mush and the herbs that were distributed with so much sentiment and success were not enough to protect the charitable miller, whose remedies made the physicians' cures seem doubtful and often useless. The testimonial of the doctor had its effect. In December of that same year a sentence was pronounced: "His Royal Highness deigns to approve that by precept it be prohibited to the same to medicate, under penalty of capture."[8]

The Troubled Story of Mangiaporci and the Revolt of the Populace of Cetona

Charlatans were not only a mob of scoundrels eager for profit, dedicated to the commerce of false remedies; many were able operators who could provide indispensable surgical needs. The arrival in a small country village of a charlatan who had experience in surgery often afforded a glimmer of hope, for very little help could be expected from official physicians, even to set a bone or assist a woman during a difficult delivery. It became a social necessity to find someone who could aid a populace burdened with "cancers, erysipelas, herpes, bronchitis, scrofulas, phlegmons, swellings, burns, ringworm, abscesses of the groin, bedbugs, boils, eczema, mange, scabies, leprosy, swollen glands, broken bones, miscarriages, sores": ailments in an incomplete list compiled by Garzoni. Often the most insignificant wounds could turn into "abscesses..., either frigid, or hot, or choleric," all incurable miseries that portended grave consequences.

The inability to work was worse than death, and country people turned to those practitioners, who without any license, performed every

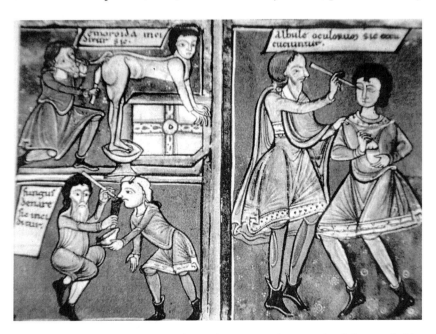

A fourteenth-century engraving shows doctors treating a patient's hemorrhoids, another patient's nose, and another's eye. Biblioteca Nazionale Centrale, Firenze.

type of minor surgery "with steady hand, vigorous, without trembling of any sort," removing small tumors, curing scrofulas and sores, excising abscesses, setting bones, extracting the stones of painful bladder calculosis. They manufactured their own special instruments: "razors, binders, lancets, scissors, needles, tongs, pincers, crushers, scrapers, and spatulas"; with uncommon courage they then prepared to "clean, shave, skin, drill, scrape, rasp, tampon, cauterize, burn, stitch, and apply plasters, unguents, and cloth strips to wounds, and let blood."[9]

Tooth drawers, healers of fistulas and sores, practitioners who fixed "blows, pangs, falls and bruises," phlebotomists or bloodletters, lithotomists who crushed calculi, surgeons who operated on cataracts, and others who amputated wounded or gangrenous limbs were amongst those operators who were able to save their wretched patients only if they acted with composure and painstaking swiftness. After learning how to wield knives and razors by practicing on animals, they were ready to demonstrate their competence on humans, in cases of necessity assuming the risk of operations that were often refused by licensed surgeons because of the danger of hemorrhages and infections. Thus an expert butcher could be transformed into a surgeon, a blacksmith could become an able bonesetter: Although ignorant of science and bereft of culture, these illegals often took the place of physicians and surgeons.

On occasion, the entire population of a village revolted against the authorities in defense of a charlatan who could prove himself a capable healer, as in the story of Mangiaporci, or "Pigeater."

During the month of April, 1766, a petition came to the attention of the grand duke, Pietro Leopoldo, written by Francesco Lemmi, the medical officer of the town of Cetona in Tuscany. The doctor called the grand duke's attention to a certain Alessandro Rinaldo, nicknamed Pigeater, "a small farmer in this territory, a man deprived of every principle of science," an illiterate charlatan medicaster who dared to "publicly medicate internal as well as external ills and draw blood, thus usurping a most delicate Profession." He added that this dangerous malapert offered a shameful example, "portending many baleful consequences," besides causing damage to the health of the inhabitants.

After a few months, the Physicians' College of Siena reacted with uncommon zeal, at first attempting to dump all responsibility on the judge at Cetona. This magistrate had in fact already been informed the year before that Mangiaporci was guilty of treating patients "by bloodletting and mixtures to drink," a serious crime. The judge, to save himself further bother, fined the defendant twenty-five scudi in "The name of our Most Holy God," adding six months exile to Grosseto as an extraordinary punishment in order that "in the future the defendant should be more cautious, and less daring."

The story has an unexpected turn: In February, 1768, a vehement protest in defense of Mangiaporci, compiled by an unidentified lawyer writing in the name of the whole population of the community of Cetona, was sent to the grand duke and the College of Physicians in Siena. The lawyer reported the indignation of the inhabitants and their firm intention to revolt against the authorities if Mangiaporci were sent away. In the letter, the lawyer described the condition of the inhabitants of the village: "[W]e are for the most part Farmers, destined to toil in the countryside, patient of Heat and Cold, exposed to the rigors of the season, and of the Climate." Because of this state of affairs "we are more subjected to ills of the Body, to stuffed bowels, failed digestion, and blood." Since time immemorial "we have the tradition, and the examples handed down by our Authors, to keep away from Physicians, and medicines so as to live in better strength."

After this preamble, the lawyer disputed the requirement that the villagers pay a flat tax of forty scudi a year, a considerable sum of money that was "not the price of merited reward but of robbery" and served to maintain a surgeon in the town who was defined by all as a "Stupid Ass." As if this were not enough, the community was obliged to pay, along with other taxes and duties, another "sixty scudi for a boorish doctor whose Election and protection is regulated by partisan spirit, vainglory, and arrogance." To make matters worse, the doctor was not even a Tuscan but a "Graduate of Perugia," who, when "summoned, leaves town, refusing to make his calls, or exhausted abed from hunting, does not even deign to visit the sick."

Fortunately, continued the lawyer, "In this Town lives a certain Alessandro di Rinaldo, Farmer, our own Mangiaporci, who after lengthy practice and profitable experience in doctoring beasts of every kind, has acquired knowledge about the virtues of herbs and the wielding of the lancet and is able with fortunate success, and often out of necessity, to assist some human bodies." The real problem was that "the official physician is jealous, and has brought him to trial." But Mangiaporci was our "empirical doctor," and the College of Physicians ought to consider his ability and the reputation that he had acquired, and not forbid him to practice the art of medicine and surgery. The petitioners valiantly threatened not to pay any more taxes in the future, stressing that the authorities "cannot ignore us now that we are a populace above the number of two thousand souls."[10]

The documents do not mention the outcome of this singular protest, but it involved an entire community, marshaled in favor of "their own" Mangiaporci, who wanted nothing more than to decide for themselves the merits of a healer without instruction or learning but with proven experience. The people of Cetona surely took into account the empirical charlatan's availability and a personal participation in his patients' problems, in strident contrast to the reprehensible behavior of the lazy doctor from Perugia and the "stupid ass" of a surgeon.

Charlatan Surgeons: "Manus Demoniorum!"

A good source of income for charlatans was bloodletting, which they practiced illegally at competitive prices, heedless of any obligation to follow the authoritative rules of learned physicians, unconcerned with obeying the medical-astrological conjunctions which they often invented outright.

They snatched the trade of authorized unguentaries, greasing those who were afflicted with scabies, ringworm and mange with their own balms. Attracted by plenteous gain in the more important cities, they carried on their trade in the hot and cold bath houses called "stoves," or "bagnios," spreading the sores of syphilitics with mercury-based ointments, imitating the "stufaroli," individuals whom Garzoni detested and described as "busy getting rid of hairs, and cleansing the life out of men in the bagnios, of which there are great abundance in Venice."[11]

A spasmodic retention of urine caused by a stone wedged in the neck of the bladder, the threat of a gangrened limb, a fractured or dislocated bone, or a hernia about to strangulate forced the sufferer to search desperately for help: Common sense suggested that he turn to someone experienced in the use of a knife, who knew how to stanch a hemorrhage, who was expert at healing wounds and sores; little did it matter if his method of healing was officially recognized or approved, or if the operator was a learned person or a coarse illiterate.

The Umbrian towns of Norcia and Borgo dei Preci were renowned for their pig butchers, called "norcini" or "preciani" for their places of origin. In competition with licensed surgeons, they specialized in operating on animals, castrating boys destined for choirs or the opera, mending fractures, repairing hernias, and amputating gangrenous limbs. With all the perils and limitations of the period in which they worked, humanity owes a considerable amount to these humble "incisores"; licenses "extraendi lapides cum incisione" were often awarded to the most able. They were so experienced that many high-ranking surgeons, when faced with highly

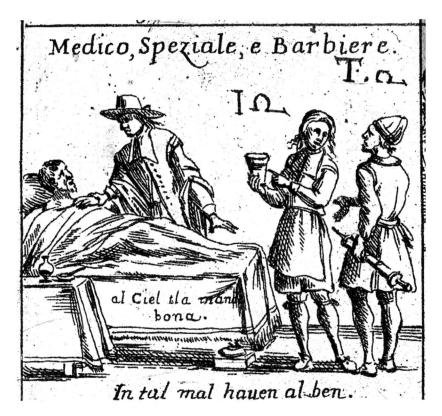

The Trio of Health: Physician, Pharmacist, and Barber (on the patient's bed a warning reads: "Heaven Help Thee"). Satirical engraving by G.M. Mitelli (1698). Biblioteca Nazionale Centrale, Firenze.

dangerous operations, preferred to defer to these wandering practitioners. In this manner the physician's reputation did not suffer if the operation was followed by the patient's death, caused by infection or an unstanchable hemorrhage.

Only Garzoni unaccountably shows no gratitude toward these anonymous, lower-level surgeons, and declares: "A norcino is none other than a doctor of testicles who cannot heal a wound without wounding." He wishes that they "would go geld the poor men of their own mountains ... for the men of the plain do not care for their services, preferring to be cuckolded than castrated."[12]

Some of these itinerant surgeons established themselves in fortified castles, others at court; the majority wandered around the countryside from town to town. Once they had taken lodgings at an inn, they would hang a chart from the door with their own portrait on one side and a list of their abilities on the other, while criers went forth announcing their presence to the public and illustrating their professional exploits.

Documents list twenty-seven families of norcini and preciani who inherited their professions of lithotomists, oculists, and amputators. Leonardo Fioravanti, who recognized the value of these operators, wrote: "Surgery does not need many things, but only diligent workmen who have good experience and healthy judgment."[13]

The hostility of physicians and qualified surgeons toward these ignorant practitioners was not so much fueled by the necessity to protect humble folk from possible harm, but by the fear that these empirics, through their ability and the favor that the public bestowed upon them, might cause a sizable reduction in the material advantages and the prestige that their own professional status should have guaranteed.

Renal or vesicle calcolosis, a painful and sometimes dangerous affliction, can often be found in the medical histories of popes and other high-ranking personages of the curia. Because of the continuous diatribes, interminable consultations and the apprehension of the physicians of the papal courts, a lithotomist's intervention was often refused or the authorization was conceded when the condition of the illustrious patient left no further hope. Pius V already suffered from calculosis at the time he ascended the papal throne. This pope, a devout and humble man who was fond of prayer and fasting "to sweeten the urinary parts," survived on donkey's milk alone, drinking more than four quarts a day. Before his death in March 1572, the Holy Father "began to produce urine mixed with putrefaction and blood, for which Physicians came in the knowledge that he had ulcerated the kidneys and bladder inside, believing that he also had a stone, from the sharp distress and pain that he felt when urinating." The illustrious consultants decided too late to entrust the patient to a norcino, and the operation did not succeed.

When Pope Alexander VII was taken ill with vesicle lethiasis, various diuretic waters failed to produce beneficial effects; a learned archiater then had the brilliant idea of dissecting the cadaver of Monseigneur Teodoli, who had just died from the "torment of the stone and suppression of urine." In this manner, using the "ingenuity of the Quick and the Bowels of the dead," the physicians were able to "unitedly contribute to the preservation of His Beatitude." In the end, a norcino lithotomist had to be brought from Paris, but by the time he arrived, complications from infection and continued bloodlettings, worsened by medicines as useless as they were costly, had taken their toll. Neither the operation nor precious prescriptions such as "Morsels of Hyacinth mixed with Powder of Jasper" were sufficient to save the illustrious invalid.[14]

In the eighteenth century, a crowing announcement in the *Gazzetta Toscana* read: "Now Lithotomy has reached the highest perfection attainable. Having abandoned farrago and a series of useless and dangerous instruments, those of both sexes afflicted with Stones can be operated in our city, fertile Mother of the most refined knowledge, with greater and well-understood simplicity." An account follows of the extraction of a stone from the bladder of an eight-year-old girl, performed by Mr. Landi, a graduate of the school of the famous lithotomists Nannoni and Son: "Having the Patient been placed horizontally, a large catheter was introduced into the urethra; having guided the wide Lithotomy through the catheter, an adequate cut was made. This served for the introduction of the left forefinger which was placed on the stone; the catheter was removed, and pincers were introduced, and with these the stone was extracted." It seems that the outcome was a success, and the operation was discussed far and wide, even if the journalist had to admit that sometimes "the loss of the Patient occurs even when operated in the most appropriate manner, and the Envious and the Ignorant are wont to make use of such a sinister event to attempt the discouragement of others' reputation, but their invectives are too weak to be feared."[15]

CHAPTER 4

"Scoundrels, Quacks and Murderers..."

Obscure Crimes with Poison

The history of poison is shrouded in a fog of infamy, of secret plots and devious alliances. Considered a reflection of darkest evil, poison was an act of treachery perpetrated through a deceit impossible to detect. Any substance believed to be toxic generated a terror that was compounded by ignorance, for the compositions of poisonous substances were unknown, and the passageways through which they could be introduced were as numerous as they were difficult to discover.

In the thirteenth century, the philosopher and physician Pietro d'Abano, who fortunately died in prison before he could be burned at the stake as a heretic, listed the ways which lethal poisons could enter the body: the basilisk killed through the sense of sight or smell; the deaf asp's saliva killed through the sense of taste; the serpent of Nubia, with its high-pitched whistle, could strike through the sense of hearing; the torpedo, or electric ray, through the sense of touch. D'Abano advised using an emerald to detect poison, for he believed that it lost its color when exposed to contamination. He gave instructions on how to succor a victim by using seven miraculous herbs, including radish and fraxinella.[1] In the sixteenth century, Don Silvio Boccone declared, with better insight, "I have conjectured that poisons inflict Death either by coagulating the Blood, or by lacerating the Vessels, or the Viscera, or by infecting the Blood or through the Venomous Spirits of several Volatile and Pernicious substances."[2]

Poison was an obsession during the Renaissance. Charles Mckay wrote in the nineteenth century that during that time Italians poisoned their adversaries as frequently as English citizens dragged their rivals into court; poison seemed the surest way to take the law into one's own hands.[3]

A sudden swoon, an unaccountable, progressive decline in health, an intestinal intoxication, an abrupt death were frequently suspected of being caused by poisoning. A simple suspicion was the decisive proof with which guilt could be ascertained, enough for a person to be dragged to inexorable judgment. A doubt could become certainty through torture, when the inevitable confession condemned an innocent person to death. Protection from poison was the principle concern not only of royalty, popes, cardinals and nobles, but of all classes. It was extremely easy to procure lethal substances from hired assassins without scruples, who acquired them from gloomy alchemists or evil witches. Special poisons were prepared and sold that could make a person die in a prescribed period; to deflect suspicion, their action could be prolonged over time.

In Rome, many young women admitted during confession that they had poisoned, or attempted to poison, their husbands; this testimony was confirmed by the august pope, Alexander VI, a connoisseur of the art. Some of these murderous females went down in history: An aura of suspicion surrounded Geronima Spara, a well-born Roman gentlewoman. In order to obtain proof of her guilt, some magistrates arranged for her to meet an elegant lady, who implored her to procure a poison that would hasten her cruel husband's eternal rest. Geronima fell into the trap and offered the woman a "transparent and odorless" liquor, a poison whose action was protracted but deadly. She was promptly arrested, tortured, publicly whipped, and finally hanged.

A certain Tufania was reputed to have killed more than six hundred people in Rome alone by selling a deadly "water," which she passed off as the manna of Saint Nicolas of Bari, a miraculous liquid believed to have oozed from the saint's cadaver. In her criminal ardor, she attempted to poison the fountains of Naples. According to the version furnished by Don Silvio Boccone, Tufania moved to Sicily, where she took it upon herself to conciliate domestic conflicts by distributing her poisonous water to "those Men who fought with their own wives, and those Women who hated their own Husbands." There was no need for a trial: "[C]losed and bound alive in a Sack of canvas she was thrown from the roofs of the Vicariate into the Street, in the presence of the people."[4]

It was difficult, and often impossible, to prevent being poisoned; it was believed that poison could penetrate metals such as iron and lead and could therefore make keys, door handles, and bullets lethal. A stirrup could transmit poison through the soles of the feet. Gian Galeazzo, the duke of Milan, was said to have been assassinated by placing a poison on his saddle; the death of an English nobleman was traced to an "odorous" glove that had supposedly been drenched in poison by the abominable Catherine de' Medici. The famous French surgeon Ambrose Paré was convinced that Pope Clement VII had been murdered by poisonous smoke from a torch. A gentleman of Forlì, Francesco Ordelaffi, possessed a poison so potent that a small amount, thrown on burning coals, could kill everyone in a room; these stories probably originated with cases of intoxication from carbon dioxide. Many poisons came from animals: The toad was considered the most venomous animal of all, yet it was believed that the partridge and the eagle could smell poisonous effluvia from enormous distances.

Pier Andrea Mattioli advised an emergency remedy in case of poisoning: "[O]pen the body of a mule or live horse, and as soon as the guts have been removed, put the victim inside." He swore that Cesare Borgia, the terrible son of Pope Alexander VI, was saved from death by this system after rather absentmindedly "Wishing to poison some cardinals at a dinner, he carelessly poisoned himself as well as his Father."

At the courts of the great palaces where princes, nobles and popes gathered at sumptuous tables with ceremonious rites, the food of the most important guests was tasted by courtiers prepared to die if it contained poison, a formality that conferred immense prestige on the personage who was to be protected. The tasting took place at a table, placed to the side, that was called a "credenza," for the confidence that the ritual was meant to inspire; the word still exists to indicate a typical piece of Italian dining room furniture.[5]

In the sixteenth century, the prince of charlatans, Leonardo Fioravanti, was skeptical about this irrepressible mania for poisoning; he was convinced that only the Egyptian asp "does not forgive." The most insidious danger can be found in "a poisonous tongue, which has more consequence than all poisons and overcomes all the human arts, and until death does not cease to persecute man; on the contrary, it has power to bury a person quicker than death itself."[6]

It was feared that poison could be incorporated into consecrated hosts used for Holy Mass. The Excellent Magistrate Vincenzo Guarini convened the most respected professors of the guild of apothecaries in Venice to examine, "with the strictest diligence," some "tiny particles of consecrated host attached to a napkin, whereby to judge if they be contaminated by a poisonous Mercurial principle or by an Arsenical element, or both." The experts placed four lice on the particles, observing them at length with a microscope. After twenty hours the insects were still alive and therefore poison with a silver base was ruled out because "Argentum vivum est voenenum vermibus et poediculis."[7] But, when some bits of the suspected host were heated on thin plates of copper, shining "effluvia" formed around the sacred morsels, an unmistakable sign of the presence of arsenic. The name of the innocent person who was blamed is not known, nor is the fate that he had to endure after the result of this dubious medical and legal procedure.

Mattioli's Scorpion Oil

"Scoundrels, quacks and assassins" were the genteel words with which Pier Andrea Mattioli apostrophized charlatans. Mattioli was the author of the "Commentaries," an imposing treatise on medical matters that renewed the therapeutical precepts of the Roman botanist and pharmacologist Dioscoride. An engraving in the ancient hospital of La Scala in Siena, his city of birth, represents the scholar with a severe countenance, his long beard in perfect accord with his irascible and haughty character. Professionally, he was a veritable tyrant who would not tolerate any interference with his prescriptions. It was dangerous to run afoul of Mattioli, for he was one of the most malicious pens of Europe. He often railed with dire threats and atrocious insults against other physicians, naturalists, and chemists who did not follow his dictates in every detail: "[F]oul flayed beast" was one of the delicate epithets with which he addressed the illustrious naturalist Anguillara during a scientific meeting.

Notwithstanding his impressive erudition, the celebrated Sienese physician was unable to detach himself from the medical abstruseness of his time and often entertained fantasies that exceeded those of the detested charlatans. He described an experiment with the strange marine torpedo, the electric ray, also called "cramp fish" or "numb fish." "Placed upon the bottom," it has an astonishing effect on those who suffer from a prolapsed rectum, for the vibrant electric shock "makes the bowel return inside when it comes out." He prescribed minced bedbugs, to be inserted up the "passage of the urine," for "anguish of urine" caused by bladder stones, but he believed that roasted locusts or cicadas were more effective for women, while "urine of virgin girls" was his preferred remedy for asthmatics.[8]

Charlatans were an intolerable thorn in Mattioli's side. The reason for this irrepressible loathing was probably the fact that for his whole life he had tried without success to make antidotes against poisons. Once, while in Prague, he experimented with an antidote of his own invention, administering a strong dose of "wolf's bane," the poison aconite, to an assassin who had been condemned to death by hanging. His antidote had no effect, and the prisoner, who was left to suffer in agony with atrocious spasms for days, would certainly have preferred the gallows to this excruciating trial.

Mattioli could not bear the fact that many "dishonest deceivers" could market their potent antipoisons with success, exposing themselves voluntarily to "manifest peril of death." He describes how they stuff themselves with fatty beef tripes or raw lettuce dressed with so much oil that "they almost swim in it." Then they take poison, "and the surrounding crowd of imbeciles and blind men run with their money to buy the false medicine ... with the same craving as when bread is given out in times of famine." Afterward they retire to a room where they drink milk all day and vomit many times. Empirical intuition taught the charlatans that fatty or greasy substances could protect the gastric mucus membrane for a certain amount of time by hindering the rapid absorption of the poison; repeated vomiting hastened its elimination, and the ingestion of milk reduced its toxicity: These are the same practical precautions that are still used in emergency treatments today. Thus, propelled by necessity, the coarse and impudent quacks, with their fertile imagination and tried empirics, found themselves a step ahead of the orthodox therapies of pompous physicians.

Mattioli revealed his own secret recipe for "scorpion oil," a prodigious panacea "that rescues from all poisons taken by mouth and also from the bites of serpents and asps." The preparation seems deliberately complicated and difficult to accomplish. He recommends the use of "oil that is at least one hundred years old," mixed with a complex variety of herbs. Selecting the scorpions is one of the most difficult parts: "[T]ake three hundred live scorpions caught during the heat of summer, and put them in a pot over hot ash." When the scorpions "sweat and writhe, add the oil, cover the pot, and leave all for three days." Mattioli resolutely guaranteed that his antidote is miraculous. Thanks to its inventor's fame, scorpion oil remained in official pharmacopoeia for centuries and, notwithstanding its total ineffectiveness, was accepted by popular tradition as the elected remedy for a multitude of ills. Venetians in particular refused to abandon the remedy of the illustrious Tuscan physician who had lived in their city for so many years; until the beginning of the twentieth century they still resorted to this hypothetical treatment, applying a cloth drenched in scorpion oil to every kind of wound.

Without losing time, quacks rushed to satisfy the request for scorpion oil by inventing an amusing and innocuous fraud: They simply ground up flies and other insects for the prime ingredient. Some Venetian chemists, to defend themselves from the ubiquitous counterfeits and to prove their own honesty, displayed scorpions floating in a vase on the shelves of their pharmacies.

A century later, the Tuscan doctor Francesco Redi attacked charlatans, whom he accused of living off the "dreams of the infirm and romantic fables." He describes how, in their public exhibitions, charlatans often eat live scorpions and vipers' heads to demonstrate the power of their antidotes. Nonetheless, Redi had more faith in the charlatans' simple precautions than in the extolled scorpion oil and, disproving the insects' sinister notoriety, wrote: "[I]nfinite times I have seen those peasants that on hot days bring them to sell in Florence, freely handle them and rummage around with their naked hands in the sacks, and be stung without the least dread of the poison." He noted that the demand for scorpions was so insistent that they were becoming scarce: "[I]n the sole city of Florence every year close to four hundred or more pounds are consumed to prepare oil against poisoning."[9]

Quacks did not rely solely on scorpion oil to survive. They often used a clever trick, described by the canon Garzoni: They would go to an apothecary and buy two or three pieces of arsenic wrapped by the apothecary in a box. The poison would then be substituted with a mixture of candied sugar and starch, so that it looked, in appearance and in size, like the pieces of real arsenic; "and with wonderful caution he now eats these instead of the arsenic, and deceives the fools ... who believe that he has swallowed the terrible poison, and wait to see if the miracle of his antidote will come true."

To be more convincing, these comedians "instruct some young boys ... to hold their breath and bulge their eyes out, grimacing and twisting their necks and changing color, having made some tight bindings above the elbows of their arms so that the spirits impede the transit through the arteries that descend to the hands...." Once the antidote is administered, a servant loosens the tourniquets a little at a time, so that "the pulse that seemed lost, and the breath that seemed extinct" return, "deceiving both gentlemen and country bumpkins with this ability, so malicious, and fraudulent."[10]

A quack would often swallow poison before the public to demonstrate his courage and his superiority over a rival, but very little risk was usually involved in these competitions. Ottonelli tells the story of a gentleman who met two charlatans engaged in selling remedies for poison in a square in Lucca. Daring each other, they determined to swallow poison and then each take his own remedy, "to prove its effectiveness with his own liberation." After taking the poison, both "swelled up"; one of them, after swallowing his antidote, "deflated, and became well with his medicine," while the other, if the first charlatan had not succored him with his remedy, "was on his way to meet false and lying charlatans in the next life." The whole episode was probably contrived ahead of time by the two cunning rogues.

"In a principal City of Tuscany," a fatal accident occurred: Two quacks confronting each other, decided to exchange each other's poison. One of them fell down dead because the other rival had given him "a piece of Toad, pounded first and toasted to render the poison stronger, and much more noxious...." Ottonelli uses this incident to develop his own moral thesis: The first quack was "virtuous," worthy of praise; the other was a sinning scoundrel who deserved only disgrace, "a wicked man," belonging amongst those charlatans who "ruin their own Souls with sins of falsehoods."

Ottonelli cites Maestro Paolo, who practiced in the castle of Collepepo near Perugia as an example of an honest and able person. One day he stopped to watch two charlatans selling antidotes against poison; being an expert, he immediately recognized that the two were vulgar frauds and that their merchandise was completely worthless. Courageously he challenged them to eat a piece of poisonous toad and then cure themselves each with his own remedy, but the two scoundrels lacked the courage to eat the poisonous meat that he offered. In this way, Maestro Paolo shamed the two impostors in front of everyone, and his fellow citizens honored him as a "virtuous Charlatan, and as a man zealous for the well being of the homeland."[11]

Bole Armeniak and Serpents' Eyes

In popular imagination, bites from serpents and stings from poisonous tarantulas or scorpions were considered the most terrifying dangers; judging from the chronicles of the time, these creatures must have been quite numerous. From Roman times it was believed that certain clays found in Armenia or Greece possessed special healing properties; "sealed" earth was highly esteemed in official therapeutics for its potent curative and antivenin properties. Galen, the celebrated Roman physician whose theories medical orthodoxy left unchallenged until the sixteenth century, traveled personally to Lemnos or Samos to supervise the collection of clays. These clays were the precious "bole armeniack," called "sealed" because it was gathered by a priestess who stamped it with the effigy of a goat.

There was such a mania for bole armeniack that Alessandro Tassoni, the seventeenth-century poet and satirist, in "The Rape of the Bucket" teases apothecaries and physicians, who, out of breath:

Ran with mithridate and Bole Armeniack
And the doctors ran with urinals,
To see what species of poison it was.[12]

The Acts of the Apostles confirm the curative virtues of this particular earth. Shipwrecked and stranded by a tempest on the island of Malta,
Saint Paul and his companions repaired to a cave where they lit a fire to
warm themselves; a venomous viper, which was lurking in the cave, bit
the saint's hand; not only was he unhurt, but he miraculously transformed
all the snakes on the island into harmless creatures. The earth from the
cave where Saint Paul slept earned the reputation of being a cure for all
ills and was considered an especially potent antidote against poison.

The healing properties of the "earth of Saint Paul" were undisputed
for many centuries; during the Renaissance, vases, cups and glasses were
made from the prodigious clay. The prevalent belief of the times proved a
godsend for quacks; clay was easy to find, indistinguishable from the arche-
type, and discounting miracles, the therapeutic effects were the same.
When Scipione Mercuri discovered their frauds, he angrily assaulted the
hated charlatans, "who sell other earth similar to the holy one," even using
"flakes of dried plaster, with much damage to the miserable common folk."
When the wretches are bitten by poisonous animals, they take the false
earth and "in the same instant remain deprived of their money and their
life."

In time, most Italian states began to trade in clay which came from
regions closer to home, with a more accessible cost. The Medici's pharmaceutical laboratory sold a rather expensive sealed earth, imported from
faraway countries. After a while, Tuscan clay, which obtained the same
results, was found to be economically more advantageous; indirectly, charlatans were proven correct. A letter in the prescription book of the Florentine Guild of Physicians and Apothecaries claims "a most felicitous
success" with the discovery of a clay from the island of Elba; this prodigious Elban clay even came in three different colors: white, yellow, and red.
Andrea Corsini asks, in his book on charlatans: "It would be interesting
to know what difference in effect there can be between the clays of illegitimate provenance sold by quacks and those legally recognized."[13]

Hard stones of triangular shape called "serpents' tongues" or "Devil's
nails," which displayed the peculiarity of "sweating" when placed in a liquid
that contained poison, were very popular. "Serpents' eyes," which were either
the dried eyes of large fish or small semihemispherical inclusions detached
from rocks, had the reputation of being therapeutic. The "eyes" were used
as amulets, framed in small medallions that were worn, as protection from

disease, in direct contact with the flesh. These miraculous charms, fashioned into rings, could even be seen shining on the fingers of many illustrious physicians.

Bezoar and Bufonia Stones

No stone could rival the bezoar, a talisman that held eminent scientists and physicians in thrall for centuries and made the fortunes of legions of charlatans. "The Market of the Marvels of Nature" specifies that the bezoar develops in the ventricle of the aegagrus, a wild goat found in India, and that it forms slowly by the deposit of light, luminous "plates" that bind together through "a certain humour."[14] It was believed that the bezoar could liquefy blood clotted by toxic poisons, an antithrombotic process similar to that of aspirin. Pier Andrea Mattioli prescribed powdered bezoar dissolved in a liquid or advised wearing a piece of the stone tied to the body so that it touched the naked flesh: "a remedy," he is convinced, "superior to all things."[15] The most esteemed and the most costly bezoar came from the Middle East. The stones, which formed in the stomachs of certain ruminants, were either agglomerations of vegetable matter around which thin calcareous stratifications formed, or else large gall stones, which were yellowish, greenish or white according to the type and quality of the bile that deposited on them. The largest and most beautiful ones, smoothed and polished, acquired the extraordinary variety of luminescent colors that so fascinated men of science.

The bezoar, besides being an antidote to poison, became a remedy with multiple applications, beneficial against plague, cancer, intestinal worms, and melancholy. "The Bezoar stone is the antidote for any pestiferous contagion, if worn around the neck or swallowed, as long as it touches flesh and especially on the left side." If the scorpion's barb is touched with this stone, "It immediately loses its vigor to sting, and putting a quantity similar to two grains of powdered barley into the mouth of a serpent with a little water, straight away the serpent dies." Thus, with considerable imagination, the celebrated Sicilian physicist Ingrassia, a ferocious enemy of charlatans, proclaimed in the sixteenth century. In the seventeenth century, an issue of the *Gazzetta Toscana* announced: "The Natural History of the island of Corsica describes the virtues and the qualities of the Bezoar Stone, which is generated in the quadruped Mufflon of which there are abundance in this isle."

With every stratagem conceivable, the shrewdest charlatans rushed to satisfy the incessant requests for bezoar. Soon, false bezoars sold by

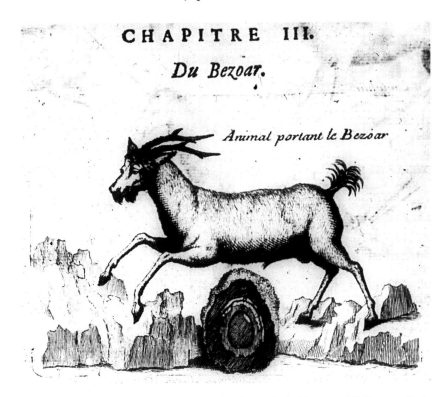

The goat which produces bezoar in *Histoire Generale des Drogues*, J.B. Loyson, Paris (1694). U.S. National Library of Medicine, Bethesda, MD.

quacks who pretended to be merchants arriving from the Orient could be found anywhere in every European country. The English chronicles were full of accounts of legal proceedings brought by royal or influential personages against traders who sold imitation bezoar.

Charles IX owned a specimen which had been purchased from a quack for a considerable price. After a heated argument, the king and the physician Ambrose Paré, who refused to admit the antitoxic properties of the stone, decided to solve their differences of opinion by testing the stone on a poor cook who had been condemned to death by strangulation for having stolen two silver spoons. The doomed man, who was promised his freedom if the bezoar proved effective, decided to try his luck. He was given a potent poison based on biochloride of mercury, and then he was made to swallow some powder from the king's bezoar; a short time later the poor wretch began to bleed from the nose and the mouth and, like "a dying animal," expired shortly after. Not even this cruel experiment was able to insinuate a doubt in the supposed miraculous properties of bezoar as an antidote for poison; the sovereign simply believed that he had been duped by the charlatan who had sold him a fake stone.

Bezoar, imported from states that traded with the Orient, was burdened with heavy tariffs. The ambassador to Portugal, who represented the Duke of Urbino, Francesco Maria II Della Rovere, informed his master in a dispatch that he had sent some stones hidden "amongst blessed thistle [centaurea benedicta, also reputed to counteract poison], in order to send them better preserved, and also to escape so much toll," in the hopes that "the excisemen do not see them." When the stones arrived, the duke's archiater explained to his students, in a therapeutical treatise, how to prepare "Cardiac salts": The powdered bezoar was to be mixed with a large number of vegetable substances, dissolved in animal blood, and then added to a beneficial dose of dog excrement.[16]

Amulets were made with bezoar; they only had to be touched before taking food or drink to neutralize any type of poison. Many physicians wore pieces of bezoar mounted in rings as an antidote against diseases and poisons. Drinking vessels made from rhinoceros horns studded with pieces of bezoar could be admired during important banquets.

Until the end of the eighteenth century, Venetian gentlemen followed an ancient tradition, convinced that it would prolong their lives: Every morning they went to the Pharmacy of the Ostrich at the Barettieri bridge, where with one "sequin" they could drink a glass of "bezoar water," water in which an oriental bezoar stone, attached to a gold chain, had been suspended.

The rare and costly remedy lent itself easily to fraud; local materials, more accessible to the public's pockets and obtainable with less effort, could be substituted. The distinguished Sicilian naturalist, Don Silvio Boccone, argued that it was useless to go looking for stones far away. For some time "the professors, and the curious of Sicily have frequently used the same Mineral Bezoar Stones" that can be found in great abundance "near the land of Calatafimini and in other places." These were large, beautiful stones, shaped like walnuts, "white or gray, disposed like tunics, or an onion, or Bezoar of the animal," good for "Malignant Fevers, Smallpox, Worms, as a medicament against Disease proceeding from rot or from excessive fermentation of the blood."[17]

Francesco Redi was not convinced of the therapeutic properties of all these stones. He found them similar to the "pebbles of the Arno" river. After trying a stone from "Malabar," reputed to be efficacious against migraine, without finding any relief, he deduced, "Either I am the most unfortunate of mortals, or the headaches of Europeans are not of the same matter as those that torment the inhabitants of Asia."[18]

The faith in healing stones, embellished with a multitude of popular legends, was useful for quacks who were eager to bamboozle the credulous common folk. The naturalist Nicolò Serpetro wrote of "a peasant, a certain Bertoldo Grattero [who], past the mere day, went to a woods called Dipachiana to cut poles to make hoops and staves for barrels." While he was working, the peasant "heard a whistle and a huge din near a stream in that valley, and contemplating from afar saw an unbelievable mound of serpents, vipers, and toads of unusual size variously restricted, and wrapped in a globe sufficient to fill the vacuum of a great barrel." The peasant ran away in a panic, but, overcome with curiosity, he decided to return to the same place, finding the same "congregation of serpents" entwined together. At the end of the third day, only a bufonid, a toad, remained dead beside a "toadstone" that "gleamed like a copper sun." The peasant called it the bufonia stone. From a country legend, the bufonia became a talisman that could cure "victims of poison, abscesses and carbuncles, flocks fascinated by the evil eye, the sick from plague; it is a most mortal enemy of carbuncles and anthrax, and conserves, dissipates, and softens bruises, tumors, and varix." The stone was given in heredity to the first-born son; so as not to lose the treasure, it was recovered once it had been digested and expelled, always ready for others. The price must have been exorbitant: It was recommended "not to lend it to anyone without a pledge of one hundred florins."[19] But soon peasants were able to acquire toadstones for a reasonable price: The charlatans conceived of a way to reduce their cost without altering their presumed healing capability.

Holy Reliquaries

A multitude of unscrupulous friars were occupied, even more than quacks, in the sale of false relics and amulets, believed to protect against disease. The friars used simple ploys that were easy to contrive, for faith and devotion made the distinction between true and false unimportant. Well-constructed publicity which advertised the thaumaturgic virtues of a certain relic was sufficient to convince people of its power against incurable diseases. The Christian world's demand for these sacred objects left ample liberty for an unbridled commerce in the wildest fancies. With little conscience, many men of the church arriving from the Holy Land made a fortune selling their own toenails to pilgrims who were convinced that they were acquiring those of Saint Peter. Others traded in tears of the Virgin Mary, preserved in precious phials that the trusting faithful gladly bought, their eyes brimming with devotion. The relics supposedly brought by pilgrims and crusaders were easily made at home; the simplest were pieces of wood and nails from the Holy Cross.

Frequent rivalries flared between monasteries and churches vying for possession of the most important relics believed to produce miracles. The most unbelievable objects, anything that had a connection with the lives of martyrs or saints, could become a cherished relic; they were not only objects of cult, but a source of prestige and wealth for these religious communities. The necessary money for their acquisition was solicited from the more affluent faithful, who were proud to open their purses and donate these revered objects to their church.

Thefts and profanations were not rare, nor were attempts to abscond with the most important relics. Thieves sent from Venice to Montpellier to purloin the revered relics of Saint Rocco, protector during epidemics of plague, were called "pious adventurers." Four heads, eight arms and dozens of fingers belonging to Saint Blaise, the doctor reputed to ward off sore throat, can be found in various countries. Two bejeweled forearms in the Basilica of Saint Mark in Venice belong to Saint Pantaleone, physician to the Roman Emperor Maximilian. The saint is said to cure headache, because he was beheaded when martyred, but he is also believed to protect against hydrocele of the testicles, perhaps because of his name's assonance with the word "pantaloons." In many cities of Europe the collections of bones, cloths, blood, veils, shrouds, corporal secretions and other anatomical exhibits were prodigious: Frederick the Wise of Saxony counted 5,005 pieces in his collection, which guaranteed a total indulgence of 127,799 years. The bishop elector, Albert of Brandenburg, boasted of owning 8,933 relics with millions of years of indulgence. It would be interesting to know how many of these artifacts were fashioned by charlatans.

There were more popular relics of minor saints at reduced prices; less potent and without ecclesiastical imprimatur, these were sold by small-time swindlers who gathered them in cemeteries. The remains of these bones, transformed into holy relics, lovingly and jealously framed in inexpensive drapes and cloths, decorated with filigree, gold paper and wax flowers, were a delightful popular art form whose traces are fast disappearing. The fact that these bones were of common mortals did not modify their curative worth; in the sixteenth century the philosopher Pompanazzi said that the bones of animals, sold as relics, had the same therapeutic effect as the genuine articles.

The irrationality of a choice and the nonscientific nature of a remedy do not always correspond to a lack of effectiveness. Relics, like miracles, were accepted by many generations of humankind; for this reason, we must believe that some could effectively bring relief or at least a sense of well-being. This is the placebo effect of any mysterious medicament: Although it may be worthless from a pharmacological point of view, often it can confer an unexpected therapeutical benefit.

Dragons and Basilisks

"[T]he Cockatrice, or Basilisk, with its hiss, and with its glance alone kills men, infecting the air with its poisonous breath and with the rays that He darts from his eyes...." This, and other details of the same nature that seem to be hatched by the lively mind of a fanciful storyteller, are found in a book written by the physician Giovan Battista Fidelissimi of Pistoia, "a person very well born, very well reared, and brought up under the paternal care of a most diligent Father, physician and philosopher. A physician laden with doctrine, charitable with all, who exercises his profession for more honest than lucrative ends." This is the aulic introduction, written by a devoted admirer.[20] The bizarre ideas of the doctor from Pistoia were not very different from the opinions that were current in his time; they belonged to that conception of a mysterious world, found in the writings of many celebrated naturalists, often permeated with the imaginary.

In medieval times people lived in a world which was charged with emotions; they were avid for supernatural prodigies, slaves to symbols and myths, and the most unbridled fantasies were held to be true. On lapidaries, in herbal books, in bestiaries, there are descriptions of extraordinary prodigies; some serious naturalists' treatises refer to a plant that grows ducks, others speak of a rare, exotic tree similar to an elm, that only grows in royal orchards and possess roots so long that they "pull up gold, Copper, silver, and even lambs and birds."[21] The tales of these prodigious phenomena were often confirmed by the testimony of travelers to faraway, inaccessible lands, where animals with legendary, lethal powers resided. A therapeutical wilderness and the fear of innumerable, horrifying diseases did not leave much to be expected from official medicine, and so imagination replaced reality and medical abstruseness mingled with legend and superstition.

"Basiliscum in solitudinem Africae vivens": A mysterious monster, part dragon and part serpent, was a beast so baleful that the price of looking at it was death. From the times of Pliny to those of Lorenzo de Medici, the withering malignancy of this horrible animal was undisputed. According to Cecco d'Ascoli's rhymes, it could be recognized by its "mortal face and glittering eyes." In the sixteenth century, the physician and celebrated

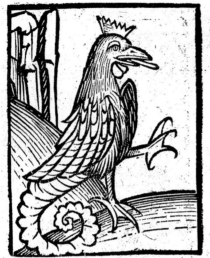

A basilisk. From *Historia et Serpentum et Draconum* by Ulisse Aldrovandi (1640). Biblioteca Nazionale Centrale, Firenze.

naturalist Ulisse Aldrovandi described the evil power of the ferocious creature in a volume of his "Natural History" that deals with "Serpentum et Draconum Historia"—a creature so terrible that if man or brute should meet its stare, they would be struck dead. The basilisk, "that suffering and death carries in its eyes," could also kill with its hiss or with a breath so horrendously fetid that it poisoned water and turned plants to ash.

This wicked creature was identified in moral allegory with the figure of the Antichrist, the image of treachery, calumny, slander, and unrestrained lust. For this reason it was wise to stay away from "the eyes and the song" of prostitutes, who, when enticing men, had the same evil power as the basilisk. Pope Leo IV alone, through prayer, was able to defeat the beast that was held responsible for a severe epidemic of syphilis amongst the citizens of Rome.

Charlatans, skeptical and unconcerned, did not lose the unexpected chance afforded by exotic legends and confirmed by the most eminent naturalists of the day. Some used their manual ability with patience and imagination to craft curious imitations of terrible dragons and awesome basilisks, carefully fulfilling the expectations of a gullible populace. By showing to the public the fearful monsters that so excited popular fantasy, the charlatan reinforced his own authority: His remedies seemed more reliable, and his business improved.

The basilisks are pictured in Aldrovandi's illustrations with a long tail and wings and fins like a dragon; horrible eyes with a fixed glare protrude from its head above an open beak which pours forth a foaming, hissing poison. The basilisk could fly with its wings or move around on eight, webbed roosters' feet. Wattles hung under its hooked beak. According to legend, there was a relationship between this fiendish being and poultry: The basilisk, it was said, could be hatched from a decrepit rooster's egg or from that of a hen which had been heard to crow like a male, a sign that housewives took for a bad omen. A cunning quack, announcing that he had just arrived from Armenia, put up for sale "an extremely rare" specimen of a basilisk; he proved its authenticity to the amazed public by exhibiting a strangely formed hen's egg, "rather long and corrupted."[22]

Aldrovandi describes two imitations of a basilisk, made by charlatans from sting ray parts: "Dracus ex Raja effectus." Bolstered by his unquestioned authority, the naturalist compares the counterfeits to illustrations of "real" basilisks; in truth, these creatures are no more credible than the ones made by charlatans. In the engravings, the "authentic" basilisk resembles an alligator with a long curved tail and a body covered with scales. This mysterious animal may have been described to Aldrovandi by a frightened traveler who had run into an iguana during his travels in the Orient. To demonstrate its "divinum partum," the famous naturalist placed a small crown on the head of the basilisk as proof of its authenticity, a fantasy that not even the charlatans dared repeat in their creations.

The charlatans' home-crafted freaks, which could still be admired at fairs during the entire eighteenth century, were an irresistible attraction for the public. Quacks brought these counterfeit monsters to the squares to be sold: Many of the amusing masterpieces ended up in pharmacies or were kept as objects of curiosity in the private libraries of noble families. With time, most of them deteriorated or were destroyed. A few specimens made by charlatans in the sixteenth and seventeenth centuries are still in the natural history museums in Venice and Verona. At the beginning of the twentieth century, one of the last basilisks was discovered by chance in the shop of a small antiquarian in Carpi.[23]

The basilisk in the Venetian museum is made from pieces of angel fish, an intermediate species between a ray and a shark caught in the Adriatic; this specimen, made by an able and ingenious craftsman from Arezzo, Maestro Leone Tartaglini, is mummified and has a prolonged beakish protuberance. During his stay in Venice, Tartaglini carried on a correspondence with Aldrovandi, and the renowned naturalist may have kept this reproduction for a time in his own small private museum as an example of fraud. Aldrovandi must have acknowledged the ability of the clever craftsman, who, with a fervid imagination and the experience gained as a wandering surgeon, had recreated this formidable monster. Other basilisks were stuffed with hemp and preserved by an ancient method of fumigation and drying with hot ash. As they were shown to the crowds in the square dangling from chains as if in flight, their appearance must have been terrifying.

For once, Pier Andrea Mattioli finds no fault with the charlatans' imitations, for he is perplexed about the actual existence of this "fera omnium perniciosissima." He cannot conceal a reasonable doubt: If the basilisk, as those travelers who have met it confirm, slays "in the blink of an eye … with its glance, or with its hiss, or with its breath, and others with its bite," why aren't those voyagers "who with so much diligence examined its features" already dead?[24]

Wild Goats and Unicorns

Fortunately, in a world filled with venomous and deadly beasts, there were animals that provided remedies against the most terrible maladies. One of these was the wild goat, an animal so powerful that it could bore a hole through an iron shield; its sexual activity was so vigorous that it "begins to practice coitus on the seventh day after its birth." A remedy known as "Divine Hand," made from the goat's blood, possessed extraordinary therapeutic virtues, especially for nephritis and calculosis, for it could break the stones and calm the pain.[25]

But none of these animals could compare to the unicorn. Gerolamo Cardano, a sixteenth-century physician, as imaginative as he was brilliant, held that the unicorn "is a rare animal, the size of a horse, with a coat similar to that of a weasel, with the head of a deer from which a single horn, three cubits long and straight, that sharpens into an ample point, grows in the middle of its forehead."[26] This beautiful animal that wandered in faraway, inaccessible forests became an object of insatiable curiosity, research, and study by merchants, doctors, chemists, naturalists, philosophers, and men of the church. Scientists as respectable as Michele Mercati and Leonardo da Vinci were convinced of its existence. Illustrious physicians such as Mattioli and Ficino exalted unicorn's horn as a potent antidote.

The navigator Cà da Mosto vowed that he had met one during his long voyages. Marco Polo saw a large animal that had a long horn on its forehead; it was probably a rhinoceros, because the Venetian traveler recounts that it was wallowing in mud, an improbable performance by an animal that was supposed to be so pure and delicate. Some even believed that God, on occasion, changed himself into this splendid creature.

In his illustrations, Aldrovandi pictures the unicorn as a shy and lovely animal as it is being caressed by a young girl; only virgins were able to

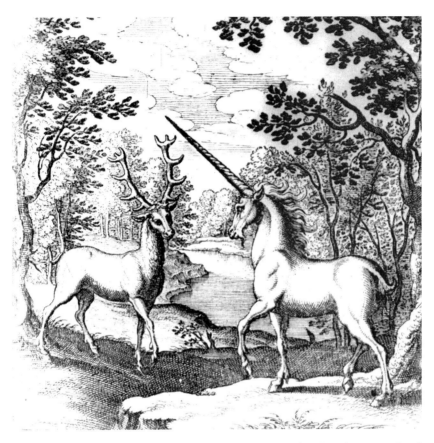

"The Unicorn and the Deer." Hermannun a Sande, Frankfurt (1677). U.S. National Library of Medicine, Bethesda, MD.

approach it. On the top of its head, which is adorned with a red forelock, is a very long, ivory-white horn, decorated with elegant spiral incisions. It was this horn that supposedly had the power to neutralize poison.

High-ranking personalities, continuously exposed to the danger of insidious poisons, had to possess the horn, almost as a status symbol. Kings, princes, popes and cardinals competed to acquire it. Julius II disbursed the astronomical sum of more than ten thousand gold ducats to procure one. Clement VII gave a horn to his niece, Catherine de' Medici, as a marriage gift. Andrea Bacci, physician and philosopher, dedicated a discourse on the unicorn to Bianca Cappello de' Medici, grand duchess of Tuscany, when she was presented with a precious cup emblazoned with the horn, brought as a gift from the Indies. This horn, a marvel of nature, "is the most noble thing that exists against poison."[27] In a pharmacologi-

cal treatise written in 1649, the horn is indicated as a "Sudorific, Alex-
ipharmic, and Cordial," to be used against poisons and animal bites. It
was reputed to cure any infectious disease and was even an antidote for
the plague. There were cheaper confections of unicorn's horn, sold in little pieces, or dried powders, or mixed with liquids. A church or cathedral
that kept one amongst its treasures often gratuitously offered water in
which the horn had been dipped to the poor. Its prestige was magnified to
such a point that it was even considered an infallible means of detecting
the presence of poison: A piece could be placed in the substance to be
examined, which would begin to "sweat" or boil spontaneously if poison
were present. If the unicorn horn didn't work, it simply meant that the
victim's fate had already been decided by the Almighty.

As was to be expected, charlatans soon had the prodigious remedy for
sale. It was simple to prepare portions of "unicornum verum": Domestic
animals' teeth, pieces of bone, and even well-polished white stones were
sufficient for this purpose. A furious Andrea Bacci storms against those
swindlers who, aware of the value of the horn, do not disdain quackery
and propose counterfeits as an "admirable medicine even against the
plague." To avoid frauds, the horn could be tested for authenticity by placing a small piece in a bowl of water; a circle was drawn around the bowl
and a live scorpion was placed inside. If the unicorn horn was genuine,
the scorpion would be unable to escape from the circle.

Belief in the infinite therapeutic properties of the horn did not begin
to vacillate until the eighteenth century; the romantic illusion came to an
end when naturalists discovered that the horn was actually the tooth of a
cetacean, the narwhal, that lives in the northern oceans. Because of its
shape, this horn is believed by some Asian peoples to be a remedy for
impotence, with the result that the narwhal, instead of the unicorn, has
become such a coveted prey that its very survival is endangered.

CHAPTER 5

Charlatans Against Learned Physicians

Jacopo Coppa Challenges the Florentine Doctors

Around the middle of the seventeenth century, Celio Malespini recounted the medical exploits of the charlatan Jacopo Coppa, who was born near Bologna and became renowned as a healer; it was said that he could "achieve recoveries despaired of by doctors" and was so experienced that he would soon "bankrupt hospitals."[1]

In the early summer of 1545, Jacopo Coppa left Bologna with his wagonload of remedies, confections and soaps and descended the hairpin bends of the Apennine mountains until he reached Florence. There he met a Florentine gentleman who, aware of his reputation, took him in as a guest, urging him to put to use his gifts of healing, a means with which he could earn a considerable sum. Coppa was doubtful: He had faith in his own healing arts, but he feared the envy and wrath of the Florentine medical establishment. He had no license to practice in that city and would surely be drawn into a long and dire conflict with the authorities. But in the end he was persuaded to stay.

A problem arose as soon as he mounted his stand in the Square of the Grand Duke; an arrogant bailiff, acting as policeman for the Guild of Physicians, ordered him to halt the sale of his famous remedy immediately if he did not want to be thrown into jail. The charlatan, humiliated and offended, decided to leave Florence right away without further argument, but his host, again hoping to convince him to stay, suggested that he petition the grand duke personally.

The meeting put the charlatan's ingenuity to the test: Bowing before the grand duke, he said: "Either I am a scoundrel, or an honest man. If I am a scoundrel, I would not consider you the just Prince that you are if you did not have me punished. But if I am an honest man, I reasonably hope to obtain your favor and grace by practicing my art in this city despite the evil and insidious proceedings of the physicians."[2]

The duke, more amused than convinced, took him at his word and allowed him to propose his challenge. The charlatan asked to be permitted to heal twenty-five incurable patients that the Florentine doctors had given up as hopeless cases. Should he succeed in his attempt, permission would be granted to practice his medical art in the whole of the Florentine dominion. Despite the protests of the doctors, the grand duke ordered that the twenty-five patients, chosen from various hospitals in the city, be taken to the charlatan. When the poor wretches arrived, the doctors held their noses, repulsed by the fetid stench of their cancerous sores, and rebuked Coppa for having fetched the "miserable rogues."

"They are not rogues," the charlatan answered, "but your own brothers in Christ, who languish in your hospitals without one of you being moved to pity or to assuage their terrible sufferings." He began his cures, "putting his skill to such use that in twenty days he healed them all, and returned them to their pristine condition, not without the wonder of all those who knew him, and not least of all the hospital assistants."[3]

A huge crowd of sick people, drawn by the successful healings, came begging for his help, and Coppa "began to medicate many, with so much dexterity and kindness, that the salves seemed barely to touch the tips of his fingers as he applied them to the terrible ulcers." By now his fame had spread through the whole city and the villages of the Florentine dominion; the "hue and cry of his good actions were so clamorous" that even the grand duke wanted to consult him about various medical arguments.

Coppa, an "old Fox, and uncommonly sly," could not forgive the malice and aggressive resentment of the better part of the learned Florentine doctors. Finally the day came for him to take his revenge. In the Square of the Grand Duke, he set up his stage, covered with a canopy "gracefully festooned with golden ornaments, oranges and other fruits," in the style of the Renaissance artists. Some large paintings were exhibited under the canopy: One of these, "A Great Ass," portrayed the court physician Strada, who had been his most relentless enemy; the other learned doctors were painted as sheep or geldings. A huge deerhound barked furiously at them as if it were about to attack. This was Chiecara, the grand duke's favorite dog, which Coppa was reputed to have saved from rabies; she seemed to reproach the doctors for not having known how to cure her. Beside the ironic allegories of animals was a painting of a huge pile of bladders, with a motto referring to the inanity of the physicians, persons with "much show, but little effect."

With a fanfare of drums and trumpets, the curtains that concealed the stage parted, and the charlatan appeared "in sublime majesty" to more than ten thousand people gathered in the square and in the adjacent streets. He held himself straight, standing on a rich carpet, holding a golden scepter, dressed, in the fashion of the Medici, in a tunic of black velvet over a long skirt of the same material. On his head he wore a large cap of black velvet and around his neck, a gold chain, given to him by the duchess.

The magnificent spectacle unfolded in an atmosphere of amusement, with witticisms and pointed jabs at the doctors who had so contemptuously opposed him. Coppa did not miss the chance to demonstrate his munificence to the immense crowd. He presented various precious drugs to the public, explaining their virtues. "This, My Lords," he said, "is the rarest, most precious preserve for the teeth that man can ever find, or even imagine in this world." He offered the remedy free to the boundless crowd, contenting himself with the generosity of the people." And then with shoving and much milling around, almost all threw money."[4]

The composition of the prodigious therapeutic balms that Jacopo Coppa used to heal the twenty-five wretched patients was never revealed, but surely the mysterious paths that led to the fortunate charlatan's capabilities passed through his sensitivity, his compassion, his kind words, and his "light touching" of the horrible sores. The secret lay in his "pity for their miseries"; he understood that he would lose the challenge with the other doctors if he placed his faith in the hypothetical effectiveness of his salves alone, without calling on the healing powers that could be created through an intimate relationship with his patients. If he had not followed the ancient precepts of the Good Samaritan, the sores of the poor invalids would have remained incurable. This cautionary warning against negligence, indifference and insensitivity is directed to those to whom the fate of bodies and souls are commended and is valid for all time.

The Pact of Recovery

The majority of physicians who graduated from the universities, nourished with a false science drenched in magic, astrology and heresy, seemed almost defenseless before the refined arts of the most extravagant charlatans. The therapeutic impotence of orthodox medicine was proven, while the remedies and treatments offered by charlatans were not necessarily the fruit of incompetence and fraud, nor were they always ineffective. In addition to preposterous but innocuous medicines, they offered mixtures of herbs, or extracts made from leaves and roots, a vegetable thaumaturgy created by popular empiricism and experimented with for generations. The elaborate prescriptions ordered by learned doctors and manipulated by apothecaries were almost always inaccessible to the purses of the less well-to-do: Often they contained powdered gems, ground coral, fragments of pearls and gold leaf — all "magisteries" that Leonardo di Capua, seventeenth-century humanist and philosopher, blamed for increasing, rather than resolving, "the causes of disease."[5]

Most doctors appealed to dogmatism rather than experience and good sense and consequently encouraged quackery and fraud. Even stern Garzoni, who certainly never felt any tenderness toward charlatans, vented his sarcastic fury on these ignorant doctors. They "jump around the countryside in their gowns as if they were a lot of excellent and famous Falloppi, ... and to earn more money, they prolong and increase infirmities for the interest of their own purses." They "think that their gown and the ring on their finger are sufficient to bring them honor ... (but) ... how many do they kill with a Mameluke's brain and a bandit's hand..." administering with blind bestiality such energetic purges that they "force a man ... with perpetual fluxions to evacuate his intestines through the main hole." Among a multitude of rogues with "murderous faces and scoundrels' hands" that treat humans like "Camels, and like Giraffes..." Garzoni remembers a certain "Mastro Simon of the worms," who, to make money, dragged illnesses out indefinitely, a doctor for whom Garzoni prescribed "an enema with ink, or broth of sardines...."[6]

Gabriele Zerbi, a fifteenth-century gerontologist, advised doctors not to be reluctant about presenting their fee to patients. The fee is a powerful therapeutic means that discourages a patient from loafing around in bed, spurring him and those that assist him toward a rapid cure. When he presents his bill, "The physician acquires more authority, he is better respected, and he will be treated with more humanity and decorum." The patient and his family will make an effort not to waste the spent money, and the sick person will become well sooner. Medicine dearly bought is of great effectiveness, given free it is of little worth.[7] Most of the populace, who could not afford to pay a physician's stiff remuneration, had little other choice but to turn to empirics' cures.

Patients were not allowed to demand compensation from a doctor who gave the wrong therapy, whereas charlatans, along with other risks of their trade, had the obligation to return any sum that had already been paid if the cure didn't work. This was the "Pact of Recovery," an ancient usage harking back to the early Middle Ages, a commitment reserved exclusively for healers of inferior rank such as barbers, practitioners of "half-surgery," and charlatans. Often this contract was written out by a notary, signed by a notable, and the sum agreed upon consigned to a person of trust. The deposit could be remitted at the first signs of a patient's recovery; the rest was given when the cure was happily concluded.[8] The Pact of Recovery excluded any responsibility on the part of the learned physician; his erudition, his doctoral diploma, were enough to protect him. It was only required that his therapy respond to the canonical prescriptions of official therapeutics; thereafter he had no fault and did not have to submit to the imposition that was mandatory for charlatans. Only if his patient did not get well, or at least better, after three days of cure, was the physician obliged to convince him to confess his sins, otherwise he was to abandon him. If the patient died, God's will was fulfilled.

A heated battle raged between the physicians who were still bound to the ancient humoral dogmas of Galenic medicine and the eighteenth-century innovators. At that time, the discoveries of the circulation of the

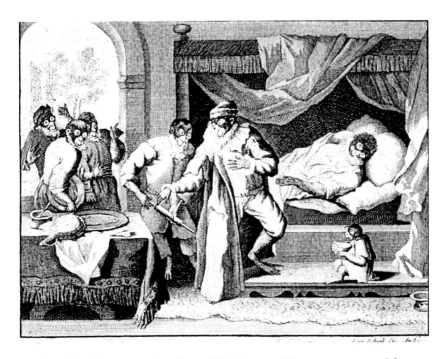

Parody of physicians: monkeys dressed like doctors giving an enema to a sick monkey. Leonard Schenk, Amsterdam (c. 1600). U.S. National Library of Medicine, Bethesda, MD.

blood, respiration and metabolism were calling into question traditional therapies such as bloodletting and purges.

The "rational" physician Giuseppe Gazola attacked the falsehoods of the dogmatists' medicine, indirectly favoring charlatans and empirics, who relied on experience and good sense. Gazola declared that "it is better to be without a doctor than not have a good one." He continues sarcastically, "what better profession is there than this, when with a simple capital of four prescriptions any one can fool the world and earn money without danger[?]" He offers this lapidary advice: "The surest recipe, and the most appropriate antidotes in any curable infirmity are diet, quiet, time, and suffering. The universal panacea is composed of these four ingredients, and whoever knows how to make use of them will recover his health with little expense and cure himself with less peril."[9]

"Rational Physicians"

The nimble minds of charlatans had long since grasped the fact that there were no substantial differences between their own concoctions and those that were prescribed by orthodox physicians; there was irrefutable proof that the therapeutical result was the same and fraud was not only or always on their part. Because of the uncertainty that dominated medical practice, it was always possible that an unlicensed healer might discover a truly valid cure. Even Giovan Battista Morgagni, the respected founder of modern pathological anatomy, a master at conducting research on cadavers with implacable precision, turned to the bewildering abstruseness of canonical pharmacology whenever he donned the robes of a therapist. This prudent physician, who counseled not to overdo the purgings and bloodlettings dictated by therapeutical canons, had no doubts when he prescribed broth of viper flesh for his feverish patients, or shrimp tails against cancer, pounded centipedes for epilepsy, powdered coral or ivory as corroboratives, neurotonics, antihaemorragics, and "little mouthfuls made of amber and human skull" as an astringent against diarrhea.[10]

While learned doctors imposed their remedies from the height of their unassailable authority, charlatans, more in tune with the needs of the masses, presented their remedies with appealing arguments charged with imperceptible but consoling hope. The people found in the charlatan, with his extravagant, amusing, and artful speeches, a modest folk hero who offered security and solace. He was well accepted because he was one of the people; he lived off guile, the only weapon that the poor possessed. Even while speaking nonsense, he used a language that delighted his ignorant

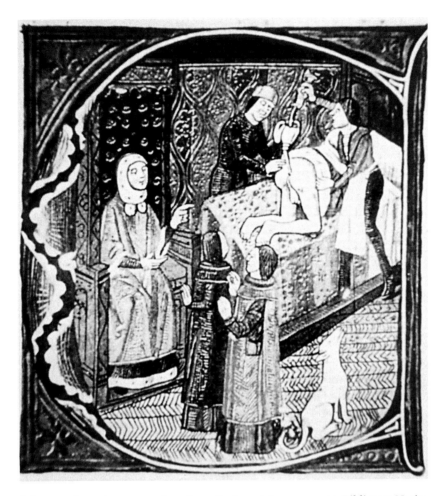

A fourteenth-century engraving of a patient receiving an enema. Biblioteca Nazionale Centrale, Firenze.

audience. He led the credulous and impressionable masses toward the discovery of a fantastic world in which it was possible to exorcise uncertainty and the fear of disease. As he stood before the vulnerable crowds who were exposed to the aggression of a thousand unknown contagions, this same coarse merchant could assume, even if he used trickery, the features of a charitable magician, a primitive psychotherapist who could, if nothing else, at least offer temporary relief and fragile hope.

Once again, Francesco Redi, the sharp-witted and cultured Tuscan physician, compared the charlatans' frauds to those of many doctors of his time and expressed the wish "to be able to undo the bonds and blindness

with which men are constrained and muzzled by those rascals, those charlatans, those quacks and scoundrels, the ignorant doctors and philosophers who torment poor Christians and make them die with ceremonies,
and pilgrims' customs and superstitious remedies."[11]

"Evil Apothecaries" and Hereditary Healers (or Noble Healers)

Not only did the vast public have no faith in medical cures; there was
also a diffused and well-founded suspicion that many nefarious misdeeds
were committed by pharmacists, those "evil apothecaries," as they are
called by Giovanni Antonio Lodetto from Bergamo, a contrite pharmacist
who, while pretending a lengthy dialogue with a physician, exposes his
wicked colleagues. Many dishonest apothecaries used foul, expired ingredients, substituting ordinary dust for ground pearls and gems, common
grated bones for powdered ivory, and local pieces of wood instead of exotic
timbers imported from faraway countries. It was well known that a large
part of the celebrated gemmate electuaries that should have been prepared
with "two drams of white pearls, two small pieces of sapphire, two of red
coral, amber, ivory gratings, and one ounce each of garnet, carnelian,
emerald, and another twenty stones, metals, woods and various medicaments" were only fakes. The poet Giovan Batista Fagiuoli, observing his
son's medicine, warns him, "If you can guess, where you read Ground
Pearls, you will find that it is lupin flour."[12]

It was considered good advice to "let all the pharmacist's electuaries,
syrups, ointments go to ruin, for not knowing how they are prepared, they
are like a sword in the hands of a madman. The apothecaries sell diaprunis,
diacatholicum, diafinicum and other similar products that are often sixty
year old refuse, beautified more than a prostitute's face, and they are not only
useless, but noxious.... Their compositions are thrown together without
any sense, and worse, sometimes they use putrid and corrupted drugs."[13]

Therapy remained the Achilles heel of academic orthodoxy; it was in
this field that it was easier for charlatans to hit below the belt. Every imag-
inable type of therapeutic abuse was regularly practiced, both by the humble quacks and the high-ranking physicians. In this pharmaceutical Babel,
even sovereigns, royal princes, and nobles delighted in preparing remedies. Francis I, grand duke of Tuscany, loved to concoct his own medicines,
repeating the same words, the same promises that charlatans yelled out in
the public squares. The duke often received secretaries of state in front of
his furnace, bellows in hand. When he was taken seriously ill, he insisted

on curing himself with the medicines that he had invented during his research and died a few days later after atrocious suffering.

At the height of the Renaissance, in a renewed fervor for learning and natural observation, princes and noblemen exchanged their formulas and pharmaceutical advice much as ladies exchanged cooking recipes. The baron of Dignola was anxious to prove that "a nobleman could exercise the art of composing medicines without diminishing either his own nobility or that of his descendants."

"The perfect Plaster, Denominated the immediate comfort of the Aggrieved," an inexpensive remedy that seemed more reliable because of the authority of its supplier's name, was made in Piacenza at the home of the Count dal

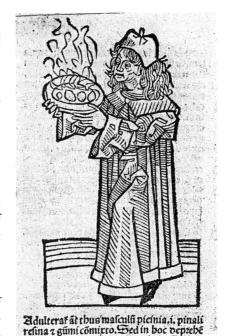

Adulteration of Medicinal Drugs. Biblioteca Nazionale Centrale, Firenze.

Verme. "Pang Oil," was a "Special Secret," authenticated no less than by the seal of the grand duke of Tuscany's workshop; success was assured for a robust tonic advertised in a handbill decorated with the awe-inspiring Medici crest: "Gemmate Julep of his Royal Highness," composed of ground pearls dissolved in wine, supplied by the Grand Duke Gian Gastone.

The Ceraulo, a Sicilian family whose name means "virtuous," were believed to have the power to render poisonous snake bites harmless; because of this reputation, those charlatans who boasted of their immunity to poison and let themselves be bitten by snakes called themselves "cerauli." Every member of the Potenzano family of Palermo, perhaps because of the word "potenza," or power, was believed to possess the ability to heal wounds. Some could cure impetigo with their saliva, or even by licking the eczema with their tongues. These and similar other prerogatives had been granted to the Vulcani of Sorrento, the Gennari of Naples, the Cencelli from the Marches and other families in many parts of Italy. The first male son born after six females had extraordinary healing powers. A popular belief held that whoever crossed the straits of Messina twice acquired the "holy hand" and could make some afflictions disappear simply by touch. Those born on Friday or on the night of the conversion of St. Paul were reputed healers. A charlatan-sorcerer, King Pipino of Mazara, was believed to own more than one soul and to possess the curative powers of four physicians.

Anyone could sell or prepare remedies, but it was even easier for religious orders to obtain monopolies and privileges. Even some physicians, in good or bad faith, invented and sold all sorts of secret remedies in competition with the reviled charlatans. "And would you believe," thundered Professor Bertini, "that even some Professors of Medicine can be numbered amongst these braggarts of Secrets ... a fact that, in truth, just to think about moves me to vomit."[14] Dissatisfaction with the canonical therapies proposed by physicians was so commonplace that not only the poor but wealthy people as well preferred to turn to the cures of medicasters; after all, the therapeutic effect, if not superior, was the same.

Specifics and Secrets During Rumors of Plague

When rumors of plague were heard, physicians, apothecaries, and quacks all proposed a countless number of preservative and curative remedies. In his treatise on the plague, Lodovico Antonio Muratori reminds the "wise judges" that charlatans, medicasters, vendors of specifics and secrets, and many other "idiots" allocate to themselves the right to prescribe every kind of medicine.[15] These inventions are born, "of a ridiculous, and reckless ignorance or from the sole motive of their own gain, with no concern about deceiving poor people who easily believe what they desire." As preservation against the mortal infection, physicians recommended cauterizations by fire and "fontanelles," cuts in the arms and thighs that allowed the "noxious humors to be artificially vented." During the tragic epidemics, people were advised to wear balls of fragrant herbs or unicorn horn or bezoar or "setons," skeins of silk or cotton that were threaded underneath the skin and were believed to discharge harmful humors and sustain the heart. Amongst the many "medicaments, Useful, or rather, Necessary in Times of Plague," the historian numbers Mattioli's ageless scorpion oil, "commonly praised by all and commented upon as an excellent Antipestilence Preservative."

A writer who lived in Venice, where more than forty-two thousand people died during the plague of 1576–1577, mockingly wrote that some pharmacies displayed handbills in their windows advertising in large lettering the apothecary's infallible preservative against the plague; despite its infallibility, they locked the doors of their pharmacy so that no one could come in, and before touching any money they disinfected it with vinegar.

A simple remedy, often sold by charlatans, consisted of plasters of odorous herbs to be worn in the region of the heart. In this "great Chaos of Preservatives," as Muratori described it, quicksilver, emeralds, sapphires and hyacinths were worn as amulets. Muratori believes that these charms protect more through the faith of the wearer than because of any intrinsic effectiveness and advises treading carefully so as not to "fall into Quackery, from which some, who make such a clamour about medicine, are unable to stay away." He had to admit however that "until now, the medical Art, with all its studies, has not yet found Specific Remedies."[16] The most reliable medicines were the "de tribus" pills, consisting of three rules: Run away immediately, go as far as possible, and return when the epidemic has disappeared.

During epidemics it was against the law for charlatans to attract large gatherings in the squares; prevention was the surest means of checking the contagion. In these circumstances, fines were heavier and applied with more diligence than during normal times. Often, wariness toward strangers who were suspected of carrying the pestilence assumed the character of a real persecution, and for itinerant traders this was a serious blow. In 1656 a delegation of quacks presented an instance to the governor of Rome in which they humbly requested that "since thank God every suspicion of disease has disappeared, to concede them license to circulate as they did before." Once the danger of the pestilence was over, the charlatans counted on taking up their activity again, thus demonstrating that quackery in Rome was so diffused at that time that they could raise their voices in protest, like any other category of workers.[17]

Tissot on Charlatans

"It remains for me to speak of a terrible scourge, that reaps greater carnage than those ills earlier described, and for as long as it will persist, all the cautions that are taken for the conservation of the populace will be in vain." With these dramatic words, Samuel Auguste André Tissot, eminent professor of medicine and physician to Voltaire, begins a chapter of his book, *Advice to the Public on Their Health*, a popular medical and scientific work that was a remarkable success in the middle of the eighteenth century.

The terrible scourge to which the celebrated clinician refers in this instance was not the return of a pestilential epidemic brought by plague

spreaders or transported by the effluvia of noxious air charged with "mias-
mas, refuse, and filth." Professor Tissot has other targets in mind: Indignantly he writes, "I speak of charlatans, of that infelicitous fruit of
mankind, whose life, so important to the State, is miserably entrusted to
the most deadly men in the world." He continues: "The charlatan is worse
than an assassin who assaults Persons on the public highway; these at least
have the chance to defend themselves or to be helped in their defense, but
the poisoner, who by taking advantage of the good faith of the patient kills
him, is a hundred times more dangerous." Their remedies are as dangerous as a "bludgeon in the hands of a lunatic." They are the principle cause
of the lack of working people in the countryside, and governments should
proceed to their physical elimination, thus furthering an increase in agri-
cultural production, the state's most substantial wealth.[18]

As a precautionary measure, he urges citizens to imitate the example
of Montpellier: A municipal edict in that city of great and ancient culture
obliges false doctors "to ride upon a thin and hideous ass, with his head
turned towards its tail." Tied in this ridiculous position, in antithesis to
the learned doctors who travel in elegant carriages, they are obliged to ride
around the city, "To the din of the cries of Children, and of the populace,
who beat them and throw refuse upon them, pulling them in every direction and covering them with curses."

Professor Tissot, mired in his pitiless condemnation, ignored the fact
that many of his accusations against quackish remedies could be applied
to most of the medicines prescribed by his colleagues: those pompous,
presumptuous, old fossils that Molière, almost a century earlier, had
ridiculed with the irony of his immortal genius.

"Doctor Anonymous"

One can imagine Professor Tissot's rage if he had known that in the
same years in which he was teaching "theoretical" medicine in the celebrated University of Pavia, a Tuscan quack of popular success with the
mysterious nickname of "Doctor Anonymous" dared to present himself
in public as Tissot's colleague. The quack's inflated and intricate rhetoric
could be read in broadsides of "Invitation and Notice to the Public,"
printed sheets that his assistants posted in every street and distributed in
public places about the city. Doctor Anonymous introduced himself as an
illustrious "Professor in Chemistry departed from Paris," declaring that
he had received "a beneficial recognition" in this famous university, approved,
as chance would have it, by none other than the same "distinguished M.M.

Tissot and by other, never sufficiently praised Masters of such useful doctrine."[19] Doctor Anonymous proclaimed that he could heal any malady with his method of cure, whose effectiveness had been observed by "the loftiest luminaries of France, and experimented, and confirmed by the University of Montpelier." Doctor Anonymous was actually Nicola Vincenzo Formigli, a cunning and resourceful Tuscan: Perhaps he enjoyed the protection of some powerful personality because he dared to challenge physicians openly. The *Gazzetta Toscana*, official paper of the grand duchy, gave testimony to his success and to the healings that he achieved with his secrets. His ministrations were so requested that a journalist assured the Florentine public, in an article on the front page, that the "Professor Chemist called Anonymous would soon be ready to donate himself to this Dominion ... [and] continue to operate, with his Specifics, marvelous healings."

De Charlataneria Eruditorum

At the beginning of the Age of Reason, a singularly controversial book called *De Charlataneria Eruditorum*, raised an important voice in defense of popular charlatans.[20] The author was not just any erudite writer; Johann Burkhard Mencken was a learned intellectual, rector of the University of Leipzig. On the cover of the book was an illustration depicting an itinerant charlatan in the act of reciting from a stage in the middle of the public way; he is dressed elegantly, a splendid wig on his head, a sword at his side. An assistant, dressed as a Turk, holds a tray of medicines; two acrobats on the side twirl in daring revolutions.

This time, it is not the usual repetition of insults leveled against low-ranking quacks, but the first assault on those puffed-up, haughty physicians with university degrees who profess a more devious and blameworthy quackery than that of the itinerant medicasters. A doctor, a judge, a scientist, even a theologian full of good proposals, Mencken reasons, "can be worse than a vagabond quack, because his method of thinking and acting, directed at deceiving the ignorant, the weak, the subordinate, is worsened by his lofty position, by his education."

The unlettered charlatan who attempts to sell false remedies from the height of his platform and tricks the crowd with foolishness, rhymes and senseless words is much less guilty than those doctors who brag of "the ability of their hands, of their fountain of youth, of their incombustible oils, of their hermetic antidotes, of their elixirs of gold, of their powdered gems, of the remedies for serpent bites, of their tinctures and panaceas, and of their hundreds and hundreds of remedies that come from the far-away Orient." In truth, what Cato said of soothsayers is equally true for physicians: "I marvel that he doesn't burst out laughing when he meets one of his kind." "The word doctor," he continues, "is often a word without significance. The art of medicine is difficult because it has no well defined rules and principles, and this renders arduous the distinction between quack doctor and honest doctor." Mencken's attack was the final blow for the category of erudite physicians after Molière had so ferociously teased their profession, exposing the ignoble quackery of a class as ignorant as it was pretentious, thirsty only for supremacy and gain at the expense of the sick.

Mencken's reflections did not go entirely unheeded, and they received a few authoritative assents. Notwithstanding the spite, the fury, and the scorn of most physicians, a few had the courage and the depth of intellect to investigate the reasons that had made charlatans successful. One of these was Carlo Gandini, the Genoese doctor who had translated from the French a book of popular medicine written by Professor Tissot. "The people," Gandini sustains in open contrast with Tissot, "will always believe in Charlatans, as long as Doctors do not make them acutely feel with their deeds the difference between a Doctor and a Charlatan."[21]

The strikingly modern opinions of this controversial, eighteenth-century Italian doctor came as a warning for future physicians: "It must be procured, at all costs, to deny the name of Doctor to anyone who has not given proof of being one in deed; to stimulate with awards, and honors the emulation to public trials of valor, so that envy, the teacher of fraud and deception, will cease; distribute, not for recommendation and engagement, but for worth ... recognize that a bad Teacher in a Chair, or in a Hospital is sufficient to let ignorance in the art grow like weeds for an entire generation of men." He made a last appeal to those who govern to apply more care and attention "to the protection of the art, and not to the individuals of the art." "In a word, I return to repeat, to extirpate Quacks it is necessary to begin to eradicate Quackery in Medicine, in which it is as pernicious as it is unrecognized."

Even if the eighteenth century was a time of huge doctrinal contrasts that stirred the scientific world, it was singular that the translator of such a famous work, written by a physician as illustrious as Tissot, dared to assume such a fierce attitude in support of the vituperated quacks. As time went by, in conformity with Gandini's ideas, the appellation of charlatan would no longer be reserved solely for those who, without learning or titles, abusively exercise any medical activity; even the learned doctor who exploits illicit and false means to appear important, to rise above others, or for his own profit becomes a charlatan. In the future, this epithet will be used as an insult that rival physicians hurl against one another in their professional quarrels, a contemptuous label to be attached to anyone who, for ignorance, vanity, or personal gain leaves the paths of scientific objectivity to embrace fraud and deceit.

CHAPTER 6

"Glorious Fioravanti, maker of miracles…"

The Prince of Charlatans

Little would have been known about the extraordinary, sixteenth-century charlatan Leonardo Fioravanti if this intelligent, ingenious man had not written eight books in which, along with tales of his many adventures, he stubbornly and fervently defends his own revolutionary ideas about medicine: an art that he passionately loved.[1]

He had foreseen the scorn and persecution that would follow him all his life: "One cannot find more malevolence, or greater envy on earth than amongst Physicians"; the main preoccupation of doctors is to "hide the name and good works of others … and this is the curse that is always with us."[2] Ridiculed, insulted, despised by the medical establishment for almost five centuries, he has finally been granted a partial rehabilitation, for his acute observations on therapy and his surgical prowess have earned him deserved recognition as an innovator in spite of his quackish boasting.

For most of his life, Fioravanti had never held a title authorizing him to practice medicine. He did not possess many means and was neither noble nor able to count on bonds of kinship with a member of the powerful medical confraternity: Perhaps because of this fact he had been unable to attain a doctoral degree in Bologna, the city of his birth. He may have frequented a course of "half surgery" without obtaining a license, but this would have given him only a smattering of knowledge that would allow him to let blood, medicate wounds, set bones, and apply, following the instructions of a physician, leeches and vesicants—tasks that were certainly not consonant with his ambitious aspirations or his iron will to emerge above others. In one of his books, he reminisced with regret that in his beloved city, "there are many foreign doctors who are appreciated infinitely more than those of their own country."[3]

Like many youths of his time, obliged to "live in other faraway countries," Leonardo Fioravanti was compelled to practice the art of medicine unlawfully, far from his native city, for thirty-nine years; in this manner he found himself in the condition of a charlatan, an outlaw, compelled to defend himself constantly from the angry contempt and the accusations of physicians.

Fioravanti's knowledge was founded on experience, "teacher of all created things." Contrary to the opinions of his time, he maintained that the physician "must acquire his science by observation," because the way to healing must pass through experience. It is useless for a doctor "to squawk theory, reason, authority all day," because medicine, "this great and lofty science, cannot be learned by only studying in books, but by touring the world, and practicing and medicating, as I have done for such a long period of time."[4]

A distant follower of the innovative ideas of the strange, volcanic, alchemist Paracelsus, Fioravanti declared that he had learned many useful methods of cure from midwives, old people, shepherds, peasants, herbalists and even vagabonds. He was never too disdainful to listen even to the most insignificant quack, because he believed that new ideas can be found even by "rummaging amongst the odds and ends of a Mountebank, a decent man who has been all over the world." Once he was in Naples, along with fifteen other doctors, called to a consultation at the bedside of an elderly French ecclesiastic who was unable to urinate because of a swollen prostate. As a group of learned doctors were discussing amongst themselves with longwinded lines of reasoning, unable to decide on a cure, a poor, lame old Spanish woman appeared and declared that she could release the patient from his torment. The physicians had nothing but insults for her, but Fioravanti, convinced of her experience as a healer, took her defense. The episode "ended up almost as a farce," because as soon as the prelate had taken the powder of herbs prepared by the old woman, he began to urinate and straight away was healed from his trouble.[5]

Fioravanti's successful healings provoked the furious reaction of physicians everywhere: They could not accept that a reckless nostrum monger, without any doctoral title, could boast of being the only one to know "the truth, entirely, of the profession." His merit was to have bravely resisted and ridiculed the abstruse, sixteenth-century cures founded on abstract, vague and inconclusive medical doctrines. In "The Government of the Plague," he belabors doctors who, because of "horrible fright," refused to cure the sick, who, "die desperate, like dogs, without being given a comfort in this world." He mentions Francesco da Lugo, who assembled more than one hundred and thirty remedies, including turnips, chameleons, pearls, emeralds, gold leaf, deer's horn, musk, goat's blood and mummies. Fioravanti ironically hopes that at least one of these is good for plague. His own advice would instead be acceptable in modern hygiene: Clean the streets and sewers, boil drinking water, and avoid raw foods.

A Keen Observer

Fioravanti was convinced that people died in despair because physicians obstinately continued to cure their patients with outmoded therapeutic canons founded on the four humors; he remarked that if a sick person chose to wait quietly for the resolution of his affliction rather than entrust himself to a doctor, he usually had a greater possibility of getting well. He resolutely affirmed that one thing is to "know by science," and another is to "know by experience," an idea that was unacceptable to the culture of learned physicians of his time.[6]

Some of his recommendations regarding lifestyle, sanitation, diet and the prevention of disease are still valid today: "Men and Women of the world can escape various and divers infirmities" by avoiding "gluttony, disorderly eating, and then not exercising at all." Other behaviors that are dangerous for the health are "overdrinking ... having superfluous copulation, for it weakens the sight, debilitates the brain, and enfeebles the kidneys." He observes that though poor people have to work all day to procure a living while the wealthy rest, the latter fall ill more often; this is because they eat too much and have to turn to "Doctors and Herbalists to evacuate that which they have eaten of superfluous and which because of idleness they have not been able to digest...." To remain in good health, one must "learn from hens ... [who] go to work early, eat when they are hungry, stay in a good humour, and go to sleep early, and they do not eat that which is contrary to their complexion."[7]

Fioravanti writes disconsolately that curing the sick has been reduced to four operations: "[T]hose that are too hot, chill them; those that are too cold, heat them; those that are too dry, dampen them; those that are too humid, dry them." Everywhere "one can find so many Prescriptions, and so many Secrets ... and remedies for every sort of infirmity, that I am of the firmest opinion that little by little, the science of Medicine will go to the bordello, and we unhappy Doctors to the hospital, for one day we will all be Doctors."

Fioravanti used plants more than anything else, one of the empirical lessons that he had learned from the more humble herbalists. He advised using them fresh, because when they are in bottles, their qualities are altered. He was shrewd enough to realize that there was no efficacious medicine against headache and that it was useless, if not dangerous, to experiment with the many senseless therapeutic prescriptions that were in vogue. He counseled those who suffered from gout to abstain from meat broths containing too much fat; to patients racked by the terrible spasms of tetanus, his advice was to lace the usual worthless milk enemas with a moderate quantity of opium and root of nightshade.

Fioravanti's histrionic inclinations, which for centuries caused him to be relegated amongst the ranks of the most brazen charlatans, were in antithesis to his character of keen observer. In "Physica," he writes on a type of breast tumor: "Scirrus, or Cancers [...] are a species of very hard tumor, as if of nerves, which are caused by a temperament of nature, and bad quantity of blood; these never come to the young, beneath thirty years of age, for their strong nature and the vigor of their blood defend them from such evil quantity." Like Paracelsus, he seems to foresee the therapeutical possibilities of a new alchemy; "for the cure of cancer, only the separation of the elements will bring honor to you, and great contentment to the infirm."

He senses the existence of other strange factors that cause disease. In his "Very Important Advice to Physicians," he states that many mysterious and incurable diseases are not caused by imbalance of the humors, but by "spirits that wander in the air, and never find rest, if not when they are shut up inside afflicted live bodies." He is skeptical of the contorted explanation offered by the doctors of his day on the origin of disease, and with his inexhaustible imagination he seems to envision that many diseases are caused by unknown entities, entities that science will one day identify as bacteria and viruses. Fioravanti insists that the medicines that doctors prescribe are not valid for illnesses caused by these "wandering spirits": "neither bloodletting, nor vomiting, nor unguents, nor other similar things." Rather than attempt to "crumble nature," it is better to put one's trust in "spiritual" cures, the compounds that will be created in the future by the bullets of modern alchemy.[8]

Fioravanti was decidedly contrary to the mania for bloodletting, sensing that "our soul" should be taken away with the utmost caution, an opinion that was in open and strident contrast with those who decreed that blood should be let for every ailment. He warned doctors: "When blood is let for smallpox, the better part [of the sick] leave for Paradise." Blood must be let only when it begins to putrefy, and if a patient has "only a little, instead of removing it, some must be added": The doctor should keep in mind the careful servant as she watches a pot of water boiling on the fire. If it begins to bubble furiously, she takes out just enough to keep it from boiling over; when the water has gone down too far, she adds just enough, with a little salt. A culinary parable that was well adapted to a rational method of transfusion.[9]

"Beautiful Secrets of Medicine"

Fioravanti lectured the conceited, haughty physicians who were more interested in squeezing the purses of their patients than they were in relieving their suffering; he taught them how a doctor should behave when entering the home of the sick person: He must seem "serious, but with a cheerful countenance, and [use] playful words…. [H]e should look pleased in front of the patient, and try to comfort him, saying that the illness is slight, and not dangerous, making him be of good heart, and good hope." While visiting the patient, he must be careful not to be deceived when taking his pulse: A contented person will have a tranquil pulse, but if he is "perturbed for some reason, the pulse is altered of a sudden, even simply because of the physician's visit; and if some man or woman has committed an error they will have an alteration of the pulse."[10]

When the doctor has visited the patient, he must examine his urine, but he must "see if it is human urine, or rather if it is not some trick, as is likely played on some doctors to test if they are experts in urine." Leonardo Fioravanti avoided these traps, which were often organized by the populace to fool physicians. Once, when Fioravanti was practicing in Rome, one of his most ardent rivals was a professor of medicine who was blinded with envy; he ordered his students to take two or three ounces of vinegar in a urinal to Fioravanti in the morning and lead him to believe that it was the urine of a young patient. But the organizer of this prank underestimated the man who was familiar with every stratagem in the art of quackery. As soon as Fioravanti stuck his finger into the urinal and tasted the straw colored liquid, he guessed immediately what it was: "Children," he said to the apprentices, "you are young and I believe you are students and I regret that your profession is medicine and yet you come to me with this hoax."

Then he began to teach them "infinite, beautiful secrets of medicine, and surgery, and urine." He reminisced about the time when he was young and an inexperienced beginner: Some practical jokers brought him white wine, making him believe that it was a urine sample from a young woman.

Tabule

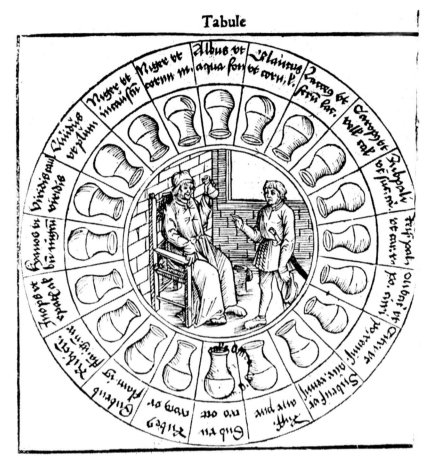

A uroscopist examines a patient's urine. Ulrich Pinder in *Epiphanie Medicorum* (1506). U.S. National Library of Medicine, Bethesda, MD.

When Fioravanti naively pronounced that the woman had a "choleric humor," the matrons laughed behind his back and answered that he had guessed correctly because "her cheat of a husband plays around with women and gambles, and for this reason she is always choleric." Refusing to be tricked again, he applied himself to a thorough research on various samples of urine; he bought a dozen urinals, and "every morning I made everyone in the house urinate so as to see the difference." He examined the color, the odor, the taste of the urine of "dogs, horses, mules, and other animals ... so that each time some eccentrics attempted to play a trick on me, they were the ones who were tricked." Fioravanti offered some useful advice to the students: A doctor, once he has examined and questioned the patient, should have his urine brought and then study it "with the greatest diligence ... because the ignorant rabble sometimes present animals' urine, or wine or liquor that are not human urine but some similar liquid." His advice could still be useful today for those who work in modern laboratories and are occasionally tricked, like the young Fioravanti, with beer or "similar matter."[11]

An Operation at Sea

In furious disputes, Fioravanti criticized the fact that the surgeons of his day were held in a position of inferiority in respect to physicians—a grave error, for "medicine and surgery are the same thing." He recalled that the distinction already existed during Roman times, because physicians "did not want to dirty their hands around wounds so as not to stink...." It was more prudent for physicians to decide only when and how to intervene and then leave the difficult and treacherous operation, which often presented serious problems such as infections and hemorrhages, to subordinates. Fioravanti recognized the necessity for a close cooperation between the doctor and the surgeon: "[I]f the fever comes from wounds, the physician will not make it well unless first the wounds are healed ... but the surgeon cannot heal the wound unless the fever has been taken away. Therefore one cannot be without the other."

When the occasion presented itself, Fioravanti had the necessary experience to treat wounds. In June, 1551, he was embarked on the Neapolitan army's flagship, ready to sail "for the ventures of Affrica," under the command of the Spanish general Don Garcia of Toledo. The valorous Captain Giordano Orsino, commander of the Florentine galleys, was at table with many "gentlemen and Captains" when a bloody fray broke out amongst the armed men of different nationalities. One of these, engaged in a furious argument with another table companion, threw a piece of bread in his face. Orsino, angered by the captain's lack of respect, got up from the table and grabbed him by the collar, stabbing him five times in the breast and leaving him on the floor to die. When he realized that the man was not dead, he repented and called Fioravanti from the flagship. When Fioravanti arrived on board, he saw that the wounds were not very deep. He administered his "Artful Balm" and gave the patient "Quintessence" reinforced with aquavit, to drink. At last, "ordering that he be given good food and not to put pads in the wounds ... in three days he was well and free."[12]

Cauterization with boiling oil or a red-hot iron, a cause of indescribable suffering, was the cure adopted for open wounds; it was believed that wounds produced a poison, a toxic substance that had to be eliminated. Some physicians thought that it was absolutely necessary to provoke suppuration by placing pads or pieces of cloth in the wound in order to expel the poison along with the peccant humors. Fioravanti insisted instead that "our real debt is to heal the wound, and not to make it rot." He refuted the idea of poison in the wound and recommended only that it be kept very clean, using calming medications instead of cauterization. To avoid apostems, or abscesses, he cleansed the wound with acquavite. Once the wound was clean, he advised to "let Nature operate, and she will operate well." If acquavite was not available, sea water could be used; "failing this, wash with urine, or put salt in fresh water, and then dry [the wound]," afterwards applying his "Balsam." He insisted that the practices of surgeons who were "destroyers of Nature" were to be avoided at all costs. A good surgeon should act like the good farmer, who, "when he sees a plant in his field that is broken or damaged by the wind or rain, he puts it back in place, ties it and strengthens it with a pole, and after doing this, lets Nature operate." Thus a surgeon will "unite the parts that are separated, dressing them superficially, avoiding deterioration, defending the region from abscesses and healing with the greatest facility."[13]

When he was called to the aid of a young man who had been bitten by a viper, an occurrence that was probably frequent in peasants' lives, Fioravanti's intervention was swift and expert. In the town of Riccio Albanese, "a man of twenty four years, whilst looking for serpents was bitten by a viper and began to swell. I had the skin and flesh taken off above the bite, I had blood drawn with a cup, I plastered him all over with liquid wax and I gave him *Bole Armeniak* by mouth … and in the morning he was well."[14] Fioravanti's empiricism was more convincing than the official cures, which prescribed that the patient be smeared with extract of heart and liver or treated with Mattioli's celebrated oil of scorpions; for those who could afford it, costly theriaca was usually prescribed; it was made of viper's flesh, which was believed to contain a counterpoison.

Fioravanti's Surgical Exploits

During the time that Fioravanti resided in his beloved Venice, he observed surgeons and barbers with passionate curiosity: Their art was "antique and noble [practiced by] humble operators but with consummate ability, without which many men would live in filth." He wrote in "The Mirror of Universal Science," that "in this glorious city of Venice there are most honored barbers, I say stupendous in their profession, who are very competent in medicating wounds and curing infirmities such as scabies, wens, and other devilry that the young are made to suffer." Their profession is of little expense: "[A]ll they need is a pan, two razors, a lancet, a knife, a pincer, a comb, two pairs of cloths, and a fork to hold them together." The barbers, he explains, "are needed to let the blood of the infirm, from the veins as with cupping. They medicate wounds, and they pull teeth and perform many other services such as playing instruments and serving at sumptuous repasts." Fioravanti admired the dexterity of these modest operators as much as he despised their habit of gossiping in their shops: "[O]ne can hear them tell every sort of new and old feat, as sailors brag about their battles, as married men tell how they were married, and how they behave with their wives, and one can hear a lot of people telling a thousand pranks."[15]

Fioravanti's obsessive desire to learn every new idea that could increase his fame took him to Calabria to visit the renowned Vianeo brothers and to Sicily to meet the Branca family. These were empirical surgeons who specialized in the practice of rhinoplasty, an antique method of grafting, reattaching or remodeling a nose or lip lost in battle or feats of arms. These expert operators detached a flap of skin from the forearm, which was kept raised and fixed to the head with a sort of bonnet tied with bandages. They medicated the flap until the skin became thick enough to be sewn, then they proceeded to the final grafting, cutting the flap from the forearm and remodeling it with a metal tool into the form of a nose. The method was so successful that some, for a recompense, offered to sell pieces of the skin of their forearms.

The technique was secret, and the Vianeo brothers did not allow anyone to pry while they operated; however, astute Fioravanti, pretending to have a relative whose nose had been cut off, managed to learn their method. Later he boasted of having transplanted the amputated nose of a soldier, reattaching it with the aid of urine, his favorite disinfectant. Urine, according to Fioravanti, did not damage the tissues but encouraged attachment. Gaspare Tagliacozzi, the Bolognese surgeon who first introduced the procedure of transplants in the sixteenth century, was said to have learned the rudiments from a description of the operation in one of Fioravanti's books—one more reason for official medicine to suspect that rhinoplasty smacked of magic and charlatanism, until finally an attempt was made to have the practice abolished.

Fioravanti's vainglorious accounts of his surgical exploits, which demonstrated the brazen charlatan's unbounded presumption, reinforced the ranks of his denigrators. Few of them believed him when he wrote that he had removed the spleen of two patients, an operation that until then had been assumed impossible.

A sea captain in Palermo begged him to visit his beautiful young wife, a twenty-year-old Greek woman, who had a huge occlusion of the spleen caused by a malarial infection. Fioravanti, flattered by the request, with irresponsible foolhardiness decided to attempt the operation. As was his custom, he had been observing for some time the work of humble wandering surgeons; he asked Andriano Zaccarello, a Neapolitan, "who in that city operated by cutting, taking out cataracts and similar things," for help. The man was a lowly norcino, or pig butcher, who had acquired a certain experience operating on animals.

To protect himself from being accused of murder if the woman died, Fioravanti informed the magistrates before operating that she could already consider herself dead. Following Fioravanti's precise indications, Zaccarello practiced a large cut with a razor, and the spleen, once the net that contained it had been removed, "jumped out of the body." Then came the most delicate part: the ligation and suture of the large arteries and veins that connected the highly vascularized organ. Fioravanti, instead of "sewing" the arteries and veins according to the usage of his time, began to make "very gentle ties with silk thread"; he then took the indispensable precaution of leaving an opening for drainage. Everything went for the best, and the patient in "twenty-four days was well." With good reason, she "went to Mass at the Madonna of Miracles." In Fioravanti's story, the large spleen, which weighed thirty-two ounces, "was exhibited for three days at the Loggia of the Merchants, so that the whole city saw it, and the glory of the experiment was assigned to me and for this all the people ran to me, as to an oracle."[16]

Later, encouraged by all the praise, he told of how he had performed an emergency operation, this time alone, in Naples: A young sailor, during a fight with a Spaniard, had been stabbed "straight through the body…" a wound, "as wide as a palm," that had gone through his lower abdomen and lacerated the spleen, which had afterward been badly sewn up by a local barber. Fioravanti reopened the wound and found the abdomen full of blood. He told several people to urinate, and after washing the abdominal cavity with the urine, he took out the torn spleen. Urine was unquestionably more sterile than the dirty pads or pieces of cloth that orthodox physicians advised for deep wounds. The patient, treated with Fioravanti's balsam, got well in about twenty days, and "an infinity of good fellows and ladies of the city wanted to see him, and all marveled at the swift and splendid cure."[17]

Fioravanti's stories were assumed to be only presumptuous bragging. As late as the end of the eighteenth century, the physician Camillo Brunori, a brilliant writer and poet, followed orthodox opinion, and wrote that the removal of the spleen is not practical in humans, but only in "Brutes."

It should be remembered that the exact topography of the spleen, its form and dimension in the living body, was discovered by digital percussion, a method that was not practiced until the beginning of the nineteenth century. The first splenectomy was performed by G.E. Péan at the beginning of the same century. Fioravanti's courage must be acknowledged, especially if it is considered that any abdominal operation, more often than not, was complicated by uncontrollable hemorrhaging or mortal peritoneal infection. The fact that Fioravanti did not perform the operation himself but enlisted the help of a norcino does not diminish his ability; he guided and directed the operation, and his method of using ligatures on the blood vessels prevented the patient from bleeding to death.

Fantasies and a Diploma

Fioravanti's inordinate boasting and his incessant attempts to commit outrageous, unadulterated frauds unfortunately obscured his real medical skills and provided irrefutable proof of quackery for his many detractors.

While he was in Venice, he sent a letter to the powerful ruler of Tuscany, Grand Duke Cosimo I, begging to be received so that he could illustrate some of the marvelous remedies that he had discovered during his travels to faraway lands: "I have found a medicine which has been searched for since the world was born, and by no other than myself has been found; it serves for all the infirmities that human bodies can suffer in all complexions and at all times."

Besides this wonderful panacea, Fioravanti proffered his secret military inventions, so revolutionary that not even the grand duke could refuse them: how "to make ships run without oars and without wind," how to "build vessels that never for any reason will perish at sea," and other stratagems to win wars. Many of these inventions are of a disconcerting naivety: footsoldiers who carry "secretly a bladder full of hotly spiced water" to throw against the foe, or an oil "with such a great stink," to which he suggests adding human feces, that it will cause the nauseated adversaries to retreat.[18]

A note added at the end of one of his pleas to the grand duke reveals Fioravanti's modest condition: He had not received an answer, and believing that the duke's secretary had not taken him seriously, he entreats His Excellency to answer with a personal letter to be sent "In Venice, next to the fruit vendor of San Zuliano…," a rather humble address for the discoverer of such momentous secrets.

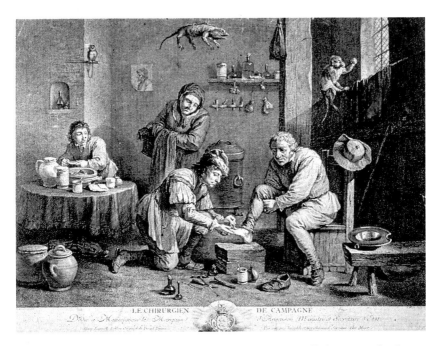

"Un chirurgien de campagne" (A country surgeon). The stuffed monster that hangs from the ceiling, the monkey and the owl reveal that he is a quack. Engraving by D. Teniers, Paris 1747. U.S. National Library of Medicine, Bethesda, MD.

The grand duke was not taken in; after many repeated appeals, he finally replied that he appreciated the inventions, "so extraordinary and worthy of being seen," but the proposals "are more easily conceived while discussing them than in putting them to use." The author Piero Camporesi notes that Fioravanti was lucky, for Cosimo was possessed of a formidable temper and could be dangerous if deceived. "To make a Prince, especially a Tuscan with a difficult disposition, feel that he had been duped, could result in being sent straight away to the unpleasant rooms of the Bargello," the dungeons of Florence.[19]

Fioravanti's insistent requests were not occasioned by a desire for profit; his lack of venality distinguished him from other successful charlatans. He never became rich because money was not his objective; he wanted to stupefy and be surrounded by an admiring public. Two physicians, Francesco Maria Lamberto and Jacopo Rasponi, were fascinated by Fioravanti's book, *The Treasure of Human Life*, in which he "promises to reveal lofty secrets never before seen or heard." The doctors entreated him to send them at least one of his "admirable secrets," along with a piece of his Philosophers' Stone. They promised, for their part, to be like "a trumpet ... that goes sounding your fame." Fioravanti, touched by their request, sent them some Quintessence, along with an aromatic electuary. His kindness may have been in part stimulated by the doctors' promise to reciprocate with some unassuming but nonetheless appreciated gifts: "four hams and a little barrel of oil, and six forms of cheese," the very sheep's cheese that was made in Fioravanti's region of birth and of which he was so fond.[20]

After a life of tireless roving, Fioravanti, at the respectable age of fifty, finally succeeded in having his fame recognized. He obtained the long-hoped-for degree in medicine from the University of Bologna, along with, as was customary, the title of count and chevalier. Even as he was about to put on the braided gown and gold necklace, symbols of his doctorate, some physicians of the republic of Venice, in a letter to the College of Physicians of Bologna, accused him of being an illiterate, dishonest quack, a false healer who even had a few homicides on his conscience. Fortunately the missive failed in its attempt, and the denunciation had no consequence, for it was recognized that it had been dictated by a few malevolent Venetian apothecaries and doctors, jealous of the success of some of Fioravanti's personally fabricated medicines.

The original document of Fioravanti's promotion to the title of physician was recently discovered by G.A. Gentili in a *Secret Book of Medicine and Arts*, of the Medical College of Bologna. The document lists the cost of the ceremony in every detail: "74 scudi equal to 260 grams of fine gold"; to this sum was added "gifts for the servants, 26 dinners consisting in a capon and a sponge cake, 6 candles for the table, 52 small ring-shaped cakes costing 4 soldi, candles for Mass and torches to accompany the rental of a carriage for the Promoters" of the medical college.[21] The tax could be reduced if the graduate took his degree as a foreigner and renounced practicing in Bologna; at first it seemed that Fioravanti had chosen this solution, in order to save money, but later he changed his mind and asked to practice as a citizen of Bologna. It seems strange that he had even thought of saving the tax, but this is certainly a point in his favor: Successful healers could earn fabulous amounts of money, but he had not become rich. "I have lost material goods," he was fond of saying proudly, but "I have acquired wisdom, rank, and honor." His quest was always for fame rather than for money. Prevention and simple cures, proven by experience and not by abstract theories, were the basic concepts on which Fioravanti's medical art was founded.

Judging Fioravanti

After his death, Fioravanti was purposely ignored; if he was acknowledged, it was only to be indicated with irony and contempt as a high-class swindler. The historian Salvatore De Renzi described him as "One of the most celebrated secretists and charlatans that Italy produced in the sixteenth century"; a rogue that passed himself off as a doctor, "an impudent fraud, who by proclaiming himself the sole possessor of science, ascribed the contempt of good men to envy, and by slandering what there was of eminent in science and morals, called enemies all those who could not approve him."[22] Even in the twentieth century not everyone recognized Fioravanti's surgical skill. The fact that he had not operated personally was never forgiven. Today, the historian Randone reputes Fioravanti as "A man of talent but with the soul and temperament of a charlatan."[23]

Since his grammar and syntax were weak, he was accused of having written his books with the help of some obliging friends to whom he had dictated his fanciful thoughts, but it is actually in his writings that he redeems himself in the eyes of the world. After five centuries, a belated rehabilitation can begin from a thoughtful perusal of these books. Fioravanti understood the importance of the printed word in the transformation of medical ideas: "Before this blessed printing had seen the light, physicians made people believe anything they wished; but now anyone can study ... and so the kittens have opened their eyes ... [and] we doctors cannot feed lies to people ... like our predecessors who made their patients believe that donkeys fly."

The first to come to Fioravanti's defense was Davide Giordano, a surgeon of considerable humanistic culture, who at the beginning of the twentieth century expressed a serene and less biased judgment in his favor; although Fioravanti often seemed an unscrupulous swindler, he was, because of his courage and imagination, the first to throw a stone into the stagnant pond of an orthodox medicine full of false rhetoric.

Other modern scholars are not entirely convinced of his medical accomplishments; although they appreciate his intelligence and perception, they still label him an astute fraud. His deceits were many, but they were in harmony with the spirit of his time, a time in which even licensed physicians competed with each other in abstruse theories; Fioravanti must be judged, as Giordano wrote, after "putting on sixteenth century spectacles."[24]

The medical historian Giorgio Cosmacini speaks of Fioravanti as "a mediator who reveals the secrets of nature so that even the uncultured can master them." "*The extravagant charlatan,*" Cosmacini writes, "must be considered a physician who went against the mainstream, rather than one of the numerous charlatan-doctors, or doctor-charlatans who must be consigned to the history of medicine as such."[25]

Fioravanti, even though he was puffed up with vainglory and presumption, simultaneously combined within himself a good doctor's passion and a charlatan's inexhaustible inventiveness, and had the merit of upsetting Galenic tradition, which was by that time destined for oblivion. Even though confused within many obscure fantasies, he nonetheless introduced many empirical remedies of "peasantish utility" and even intuitively glimpsed the discoveries of a future science. Had this intelligent healer lived in our times, he would have been a controversial standard bearer of alternative medicine. When he wrote that a doctor must "cure the infirmity, that is, the effect of the cause, and not the cause [for] if this cannot be cured, it is not necessary to know it," he seemed an illuminated precursor of the theories of homeopathic medicine.

If Fioravanti's ghost were to glance these days at the window of an eighteenth-century pharmacy in Via Condotta, a narrow street in the ancient center of Florence, it would be surprised to see a small, dark bottle. The label reads "Fioravanti's Balm." Venetian turpentine, galbanum, storax, bayberries, zedoary, cinnamon, nutmeg, and fraxinella are the principal drugs in the concoction, which can be used as a bland revulsive, a fragrant mixture diluted in a strong alcoholate. Fioravanti prescribed it for wounds, as an antidote against the poison of abscesses. So that a larger amount would be consumed, he ordered that the patient be massaged all over the body. The balm, after almost five centuries, is inevitably destined to soon disappear, supplanted by more potent, but less aromatic, compounds created by modern pharmochemistry.

Fioravanti is still being discussed and judged. It is a difficult task, for he sums up within himself the personalities of a charlatan, an impostor, a cautious healer, a dauntless surgeon and an illuminated therapist. But the ancient Persian root of the word "medicus," that title for which Fioravanti so yearned, incorporated the ambiguous meanings of healer and sorcerer.

CHAPTER 7

The Feverish Search
for a Remedy

Dreams, Hopes, and Unfulfilled Expectations

"There are only a few small carafes of my portentous Elixir left....
[H]ere is the wondrous center of all knowledge in theoretical and practical medicine! Here is the Hundred Years Life, the Everlasting, the veritable Perpetuator of Health. It is the quintessence of a hundred simples, of
two hundred salts, of three hundred alkali, of four hundred metals, of five
hundred earths, of six hundred fires, of seven hundred gasses, of eight
hundred acids, of nine hundred 'rheumatical' plants, and of a thousand
vital spirits, volatile and quadruped. This is the real water, the real wine,
the real oil, the real vinegar, the real prune, the real balm, the real fluid,
the real plaster, the real unguent.... Inside and outside it relieves: fevers,
migraines, afflictions of the eyes, the nose, the ears, the mouth, scurvy,
incarcerated and 'extra carceres' hernia, angine, sore throat, pleurisy,
fluxions and refluxions, colics, lack of appetite, gluttony, bad air, colic,
epilepsy, conflicts with mother or father, difficult childbirth, scabies, ringworm, leprosy, acne, bubos...."[1] The charlatan Gambalunga, engrossed in
the emphatic sale of his remedy, utters this nonsense as he looks down from
his platform. How can we disagree with this "archblusterer of medicine"
when he declares that the remedy is the only solution for the infinite
afflictions of our bodies?

A remedy is the gift that is expected from medicine: a wondrous material or metaphysical entity that will correct the functions of the body, combat pain, subdue sickness, or at least gain time in the hope that the healing
forces of nature will do their job. The search for a remedy has absorbed

humankind in every period of its history. One of the most ancient Chinese legends tells of the Emperor Shen-Nung, 2800 years before Christ, who had his stomach replaced with a glass phial so that he could try out on himself some medicinal plants that he had discovered and show their stupendous virtues to his people.[2]

The history of remedies is an interminable succession of dreams, false hopes, unfulfilled expectations, laborious attempts, vain efforts, blunders and withering disappointments: a terrain easily conquered by evil frauds, counterfeiters, able cheats and swindlers attracted by the mirage of effortless gain or the narcissistic desire to achieve fame and prestige.

The science of remedies followed far behind other branches of medicine; therapy has always been the "soft underbelly," where quackery was able to strike with ease. Jean Jacques Rousseau was led to comment: "[I]n no other field of human thought can so much superstition and so much quackery be found as in the art of inventing and using remedies."

In times when the treatment of diseases dwelled in the realm of uncertainty or absolute error, and medicines prescribed by learned doctors were of no use, the ingenuity of charlatans took the upper hand. If a magisterial drug seemed to produce a tangible effect, if one of the many remedies ordered by orthodox doctors created hope or faith in the minds of the people, they quickly rushed to create an imitation which usually had the same effect as the original drug: Thus the therapeutic science of physicians was rendered ever more worthless and uncertain.

Popes and Gems

For centuries there was the conviction that the more a drug was precious, costly and rare, the more it was efficacious. At the beginning of the thirteenth century, Marbot, the influential bishop of Rennes, listed the curative potential of sixty precious stones in a book that was widely read. "Diamargariton," a potent electuary, is described in the alchemical recipes of Guillaume Fabri de Die, the physician of Amadeus VIII of Savoy: It is composed of gold, hyacinths, pearls, sapphires, emeralds, amber, and coral.[3] "Very precious waters and oils" were invented and prepared in the Medici foundry. A French culinary document gives the recipe for the "Restorative of Chiquart," a useful therapy for delirium and loss of memory, a remedy that chefs prepared by putting two flasks, one inside the other, over a slow fire: The outer one was stuffed with chicken, the inner one with precious gems.

Nicolas Copernicus earned the title of doctor in medicine at the University of Padua and for a long time owed his fame more to medicine than to the study of celestial objects. High-ranking political and religious personalities were amongst the patients that he treated, sometimes by correspondence. At the same time he offered his knowledge free to the poor, not wanting to "leave them at the mercy of medicasters and charlatans." A medical prescription written in his hand, forgotten amongst the pages of his annotations on the "Elements' of Euclide," was found preserved in the library of Uppsala. In the recipe, along with chamomile, lemon, and cinnamon, the great scientist carefully measures in drachmas and "scruples," doses of ground sapphires, grated deer's horn, powdered silver, pearls, and emeralds. The man who revolutionized the theories of the solar system, who defied every dogma that put the earth at the center of the universe, lacked the courage or the critical intuition to argue with the insane precepts that were part of the extravagant and fanciful therapeutics of his age.[4]

Petrus Hispanus, the physician who became Pope John XXI and in 1277 tragically perished beneath the collapsed ceiling of the apostolic palace in Viterbo, was more cautious. On the first page of his "Thesaurum Pauperum," a collection of popular remedies compiled for the poor, the august author invokes for his reader: "God help thee!"—a wish that is timely for all who fall ill, in any age.

During the night of Saturday, February 15, 1605, the Aldobrandini pope, Clement VIII, was stricken with a grave apoplectic stroke, caused, according to his archiater, by "a great profusion of catarrh trickling from his head and brain in the form of drops." After repeated and excruciating cauterizations with a hot "button iron," it was decided to insert the poor pontiff's head "into the viscera of a gelded lamb," a "sympathetic" cure that, in the physicians' account, obtained a miraculous effect for only a few moments; the patient soon worsened to such a point that they were forced to attempt other remedies. It was considered essential to use medicines that were rare and beyond the reach of common mortals; doctors tried every means available to treat the illustrious patient, administering potable gold and other vital broths made of pearls and ingredients of "value each one up to two hundred scudi, opening his mouth by force." The same fate befell Clement VII, compelled, while already dying, to gulp down three thousand ducats worth of powdered diamonds. The serious renal-vesical calculosis that brought Gregory XIV to rapid death was treated with ground gold and gems, a therapy that elicited from the historian Ludovico Antonio Muratori the comment, "[T]his good Pope was surrounded by either some very silly physicians or some very clever thieves."[5]

The papal chronicles narrate that in the summer of 1676, Clement X developed an uncontrollable diarrhea which his doctors pronounced due to "dropsy or malignant fever." The powerful archiater, Florido Salvatore, tried to cure him with extract of coral, but without success. The pope's nephew, a cardinal, suspected the therapy of being the cause of his uncle's death, a loss so ruinous for him that he vented his rabid fury on the physician with blows and kicks.[6]

The mortal bodies of pontiffs often became experimental terrain for new and expensive medicines, for the illness of a pope was cause for religious and political consternation. The large circle of physicians that surrounded His Holiness was continuously urged by concerned relatives and courtiers to use any available means to repair the infirmities of old age and combat the ailments of the venerable old men; the strangest remedies and the most recondite therapies were tried on the bodies of these eminent patients, almost always causing unbelievable suffering instead of giving even temporary relief. It was the conviction of many celebrated archiaters that a sick pope could not be treated with vegetable compounds recommended by herbalists and charlatans; yet, if they had used those simple, empirical remedies, they could perhaps have procured a beneficial palliative effect, and at the very least saved a considerable amount of money.

The Philosopher's Stone and Potable Gold

Alchemy offered quacks an unexpected chance. Leonardo di Capua voiced his concern in 1681, writing that "the arrogance of our Century … is known by the abuse of badly fabricating, or rather roughly making, chemical remedies, which one sees publicly used by Quacks, by Charlatans, and by the lowest women, who sell them in heaps on their benches, and during fairs." Di Capua noticed that these false remedies, copied to perfection, were so ubiquitous that "often they can be bought at the apothecaries, and by doctors who then dispense them to their patients."

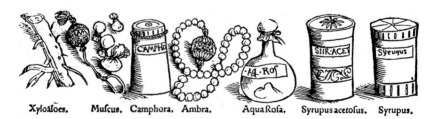

Xyloaloes.   Mufcus.   Camphora.   Ambra.   AquaRofa.   Syrupus acetofus.   Syrupus.

Fundamental Herbal Medicines. Ibn Butlan in *Tacuini Sanitatis,* J. Schottum (1531). U.S. National Library of Medicine, Bethesda, MD.

In his book, "On the Uncertainties of Medicines," this adversary of chemical remedies, heedless of universal censure, concluded that the real science of drugs is nonexistent; it is none other than "an illusion and a desire."[7]

For centuries, erudite medicine's most ardent hopes were placed on the discovery of a universal remedy. Roger Bacon reminisced that "sages and great philosophers of ancient times have taught us that many glorious and worthy medicines can be drawn from wine, precious stones, oils, vegetables, minerals, and animals; but the most precious of medicines, the mother of philosophers and the prince of remedies, is the quintessence, the philosopher's stone or elixir of life: a medicine that prolongs human life beyond its natural end, that sustains man in health, in natural virility of the body and mind, in clearness of memory and sharpness of intellect."

While alchemists toiled over their alembics in the spasmodic search for this admirable quintessence, another fine remedy was available for those who could afford it: gold, the terrestrial representative of the celestial sun, the universal medicament, the panacea that could provide all the vital energies. It was recommended to nourish oneself with potable gold, or to add the noble metal to tinctures, syrups, and electuaries, or apply it to the skin in thin sheets over the stricken organ.

The historian and pharmacologist Alberico Benedicenti wrote that "Some diluted gold in turpentine, thus fabricating potable angelic gold; after treating this liquid, a gold lime known as 'fulminating' was obtained, and this was treated with the spirit of the urine of a healthy man addicted to wine; it sold for a hefty price in London with the name of 'potable gold of brother Anthony,' and was exported to France and Germany."[8] By this time anyone who declared himself expert in medicine or chemistry could propose his own method for treating gold and provide therapeutical instructions.

Leonardo Fioravanti declared "a medicine can be made with the sun that we call gold that will nearly give life to the dead." If a remedy is desired that "removes grave infirmities from this fragile life ... this is potable gold, over which philosophers have discussed so much, stating that breath returns to the dead."[9] His prescription was to stuff ten chickens with thin sheets of the purest gold, and after cooking them for thirty hours over a slow fire, to drink the dense broth. With cunning intuition, he realized that the hearty chicken broth was worth more as a tonic than the golden metal.

Gerolamo Cardano, a celebrated physician of the sixteenth century, recommended adding gold to boiled, uncleaned hens, so as to gulp down their fetid excrements more easily.[10]

While physicians confessed themselves at a loss to cure the sores of leprosy and syphilis, the empirical charlatans correctly guessed that the same remedy that they used with success against scabies could be employed against these repugnant diseases. An amused Girolamo Fracastoro, the physician who gave syphilis its name, told of a friend, a charlatan who had the idea of using mercury as a cure for the disease; when he spoke to some doctors about it, they laughed in derision, and the poor man, intimidated, changed the subject. Later, other doctors took up the idea and made a fortune. Over time, mercurial cures in ever larger doses were transformed into infernal and murderous treatments. The physician Bovio chastised mercurialists with these words: "[T]hey oil the miserable infirm with live mercury mixed with pork suet, making their mouths become sore, their teeth fall out, their gums and palate rot, and their eyes, palates, noses, and mouths pour forth torrents of putrid humors, corrupt catarrhs, and anguished slaver. Surely ninety die, and the other ten remain perpetually sick." A story circulated about a Parisian merchant who was so soaked with mercury that when he touched gold coins, they turned to silver!

"Ignobilia et Indigna"

From ancient times, medical practitioners did not disdain to prescribe remedies that were made from excrement; it was believed these were the body's emissaries and that they contained the qualities and talents of their original owners. Nothing of the human reserve was to be wasted: urine, saliva, sweat, smegma, sperm, milk and blood all figured as ingredients in official therapeutics.[11]

Human feces were the most prized, but official medical prescriptions often contained feces of dogs, hens, pigs, and peacocks: These last were particularly preferred because they were supposed rich in volatile salts. The Sienese doctor Pier Andrea Mattioli thought that fresh human feces "removed swelling from wounds" and could be of "notable virtue for sore throat." He agreed with Galen that the excrements of children, nourished with lupine and old wine, were the best, "because the feces that are generated do not stink." He advised drinking the water produced in a steaming alembic filled with human excrements, "especially those of a redheaded man," to cure fistulas, corrosive ulcers, and ringworm. He also recommended a generous drink of this water for "spots and cataracts of the eyes and for cancers ... the excrements of goats, drunk in wine and bile, bring on menstruations and childbirth, those of wild boar chopped in vinegar or wine arrest bloody sputum, those of large rats, put into suppositories for children, make them evacuate their bowels."[12] This "sulfur mirabilis," as Paracelsus called it, did not appear in the concoctions that charlatans proposed; they only used it to prepare practical jokes to amuse their public.

Urine, even more than blood, was one of the curative and diagnostic pillars of humanity. The physician Soleandro generously gave his own healthy urine to patients afflicted with oppilation of the liver or spleen. Toward the Renaissance, urine became steadily more fashionable. Those who suffered from gout could alleviate their pain by drinking the wonderful golden fluid; wind in children could be cured with urine enemas; pregnant women were instructed to drink their husbands' urine for a fortunate delivery; eunuchs' urine rendered women fertile, and that of young girls was an antidote against poisonous serpent bites. A glass of "water of wildflowers," the poetic name given to cow urine, was an excellent defense against intestinal ailments if drunk in the morning on an empty stomach.

A celebrated, sixteenth-century scholar of metabolism, Santorio Santorio from Capodistria, invented a special apparatus with which he could give himself an enema with his own warm urine, in the belief that it stimulated intestinal peristalsis. A century later, the academic and physician Bernardino Ramazzini from Padua recalled how young nuns, suffering from irregular menstruations, were cured by drinking urine, an empirical demonstration of the potency of the hormonal substances that were contained in the liquid.[13] In the eighteenth century, urine was believed to indicate one's state of health. Brunner, a French doctor, announced that this "daughter of blood is the genuine Compass of Medicine." The eminent English doctor Sir William Guld was convinced that the famous Greek maxim "Know thyself" was to be interpreted as an invitation to know one's own urine.

Many works of art recall to memory one of the most frequent symbols of ancient diagnostics: the picture of the physician examining a flask of a patient's urine against the light in order to observe its transparency and color, or in the act of tasting it to ascertain the presence of sugar.

Uroscopy, which could have provided empirically useful diagnostic information, became for the most part a mystificatory practice, a form of divination in which it was difficult to distinguish a cheating doctor from a cunning charlatan. In eighteenth-century Europe there was a plethora of "piss doctors," an army of specialists who promised that they could recognize more than ten types of clear urine and perhaps hundreds of kinds of cloudy urine. These crafty uroscopists, always occupied in interminable discussions and fantasies, decided that the patient's presence was no longer

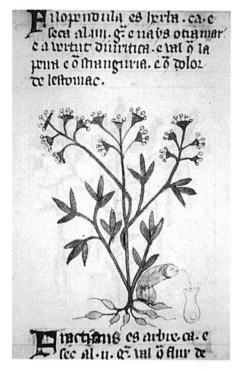

A fourteenth-century drawing of dropwort (*Filipendula hexapetala*), a plant used for urinary complaints. Near the root a penis is urinating into a bottle. Biblioteca Nazionale Centrale, Firenze.

necessary: A flask of urine was sufficient for a diagnosis and the prescription for the cure; the doctor could avoid annoying meetings with the sick. "Bring me your urinal and I will see within the disease," was their motto.[14]

In a letter conserved in the Medici archives, Carlo Gondi, a Florentine abbot who resided in France, reported the wonderful cures of a doctor of Boeuf who sent his servants out to "bring every day by carriage the flasks of urine that are sent to him." Such was the fame of this French doctor that guards were necessary to keep the crowds at bay.[15]

The public was advised not to throw their urine away: The broadsides posted by uroscopists announced, "with only a few coins everyone can obtain an analysis suited to the discovery and prevention of many terrible diseases." There were a few attempts to rebel against this urino-divinatory mania at the beginning of the nineteenth century: "[I]nstead of sending one's urine to these piss prophets," wrote an anonymous sage, "it would be better to throw it in their faces!"

Sometimes wicked tricks were played on the doctors who examined urine samples. The practical jokes prepared with false urine were legion: A German charlatan named Mayerbach sent a sample of cow urine to a physician who replied that it belonged to "a woman in a state of acute sexual enjoyment." In the story of "Lu prenu di Murriali" ("The Pregnant Man of Monreale"), the diagnostic capacities of a uroscopist were put to the test when a pregnant woman by mistake sent her own urine to the doctor instead of that of her sick husband. The amazed examiner emitted a diagnosis of extraordinary pregnancy in a man.

Finally, at the beginning of the nineteenth century, a "Medicamentorum officinalium Censura," indicated which officinal remedies were to be eliminated as therapies: Amongst these were the "ignobilia et indigna," such as hooves of elk, horses, and so on, and those of a "sordid and nauseous" nature such as extract of human skull and excrements.[16]

Powerful remedies could be extracted from blood: The Franciscan monk Domenico Auda, chief apothecary of the Roman hospital of Santo Spirito, one of the most celebrated laboratories of the sixteenth century, revealed a magnificent secret for the distillation of the quintessence of human blood, a composition that was copied from the "magna medicina" with which Fioravanti, a century earlier, had "almost resuscitated the dead." The apothecary declared that after interminable distillations of blood he had obtained the "quintessence of fire, of earth, and of water." Of these, only fire contains the "marvelous force." "If one were to be found on the point of death, and had lost his speech, by giving him the quantity of a chickpea (of this precious element) dissolved in a little wine and procuring thus to have him swallow it immediately, he will come to himself, and at least for an hour he will speak, and can adjust his affairs."[17]

Auda suggested that it was better to have this quintessence circulate in horse manure in order to bring it to "supreme perfection," a "perfection" that Fioravanti looked down upon, having grasped the fact that any quintessence that would wake the dead had to be based mainly on the corroborative action of a potent aquavit. With this he could truly "resuscitate the dead, but only those abandoned by doctors, the ones that God did not yet want to call unto Himself."[18]

A Case of Hydrophobia

Early in the morning on the twentieth of July, 1842, an elegant carriage halted in front of the main door of the Royal Hospital of Santa Maria Nuova in Florence. The most prestigious hospital in the city, it had been founded in the thirteenth century by Monna Tessa, the devout nursemaid of Dante's Beatrice Portinari. Greeted with profound respect by the ushers, the superintendent of the hospital, His Excellency, Prince Louis Lumano Bonaparte of Canino, mounted the stairway to the council chamber on the second floor where the chief physician and ten illustrious professors of medicine and surgery awaited him. The reason for a meeting at this unusual hour was the urgent necessity to know His Excellency's opinion regarding a pressing clinical matter of particular interest: the choice of treatment to be administered to a young man who had been brought to the hospital in critical condition.

The details were painstakingly reported in the *Medical and Surgical Gazette* of the Florentine Medical Society of February 15, 1843: A fifteen-year-old boy, Luigi Grassini, had been bitten on the hand by a mastiff dog a month earlier. Sometime afterward, the boy had felt acute pain in his hand and arm and exhibited a "clenching constriction of the jaws," a frightening clinical picture that referred, without the slightest doubt, to hydrophobia. After entering the hospital, the boy's condition had worsened from day to day; not even the slightest improvement was noticed following a symptomatic therapy based on mustard plasters and enemas of barley water and morphine.

In the heated consultation that took place amongst the twelve illustrious luminaries, the prevalent opinion was that viper venom should be used in the attempt to save the stricken boy. Almost all of the professors, who still adhered to the ancient precepts of Galen, agreed that this cure was the only means with which they could hope to obtain "a mitigation of the phenomena [*sic*] of hydrophobia." Invoking the principle "ad juvantibus et ledentibus," with the consent of Prince Bonaparte and notwithstanding Professor Enrico Burci's lone contrary vote, the decision was reached to introduce viper poison into the patient's body. Nine excited and famished vipers, provided by the hospital pharmacy, were put under the sheets around the unfortunate patient's legs. The cold clinical report states that "after four hours of delirium and convulsions, the boy, crying out his mother's name, expired."[19]

A high level scientific discussion was kindled by this tragic death, which was certainly provoked, or at least hastened, by the questionable therapeutic intervention. According to some professors, the dose of poison administered was insufficient; for others the viper poison had failed to work because it had not been given soon enough after the dog bite. Prince Bonaparte, an expert chemist and naturalist, delivered a learned disquisition on the curative properties of echidnine, the scientific name of viper poison. The conclusion was reached that in future cases of hydrophobia, it would be more expedient to inject viper poison directly into the patient's veins.

Was it irresponsible ignorance, pompous presumption, or the eagerness to try out a dangerous experiment that had so insanely deflected the intellects of these eminent physicians? This homicidal treatment, attempted in the middle of the nineteenth century, in one of the most famous hospitals in Italy, only a few years before the discovery of a rabies vaccine, seems incomprehensible in our day, but at that time the use of viper poison was still considered a method worthy of respect. Viper flesh had been for centuries the main and fundamental ingredient of the most celebrated remedy in the history of medicine.

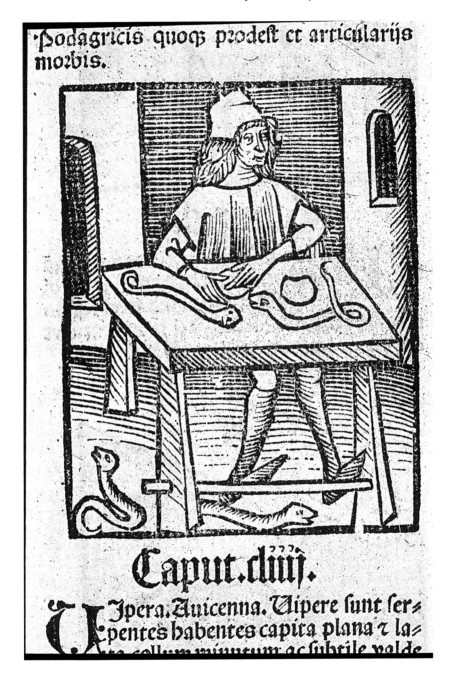

The preparation of viper flesh (1500). Biblioteca Nazionale Centrale, Firenze.

Theriac: A Prestigious Brew

No drug created by humans has ever lasted, or perhaps will ever last, for as long a time as theriac. Theriac was a colossal brew, a prodigious mixture containing, along with viper flesh, substances of every type, created by congregations of learned academics, jealously prepared and guarded like a treasure, believed to be the most powerful and universal remedy on earth. In the history of remedies, only one other drug was able to rival theriac or attain the same success; this was orvietan, a remedy that was entirely conceived by the fanciful minds of charlatans.

Error, ignorance, pedantry, deceit and suggestion contributed to preserve these two great remedies; their incredible history, if nothing else, demonstrates how, in the art of creating and dispensing remedies, medicine and quackery have walked hand in hand over the ages.

Theriac was made of hundreds of ingredients of all kinds, commonplace and familiar or rare and precious. Its fame was so widespread that the word became synonymous with panacea, a drug that was useful for all maladies. In reality, it was a medicine that, though fortunately harmless, was totally inefficacious, but which nonetheless must have somehow aroused a reaction in bodies and spirits. Authorities and governments threatened severe penalties for any attempt at forgery, and the most celebrated academics kept careful vigil over its manufacture. The remedy's elaborate composition, the obsessive search for the most exotic and costly ingredients, the vast expenditures necessary for its fabrication, the sumptuous public ceremonies for its preparation became affairs of state. For the powerful guilds of physicians and apothecaries, for the universities of every state from Genoa to Florence, from Bologna to Rome, to Naples, to Salerno, and as far as the kingdom of Sicily, the production of theriac symbolically represented cultural and commercial supremacy. The Serene Republic of Venice took the lead: The production of the drug, regulated by rigid laws, was carried out by the best apothecaries under the supervision and control of magistrates and physicians.

The creation of the first viperine theriac is credited to Andromacus, Nero's physician; keenly concerned, not without reason, that the emperor could be poisoned, he used the flesh of the poisonous viper as the principle ingredient. The Romans took theriac not only as a curative drug, but as a prevention against disease, much as vaccinations are practiced today. The Roman ships that arrived from Egypt were often loaded with deadly reptiles. Scribonio Largo advised travelers who were departing on expeditions to faraway lands to take the remedy along with them for the trip.

The distinguished, seventeenth-century anatomist and surgeon

Marco Aurelio Severino recommended eating capons that had been slain by vipers. Celebrated academics such as Aldrovandi, Malpighi and Ramazzini succumbed to the fame of theriac, even prescribing it for scabies. Giovan Battista Morgagni had complete faith in viper flesh. His prescription for a three-year-old girl afflicted with diarrhea reads: "half a mountain viper in condensed broth."

"There was such faith in the effects of theriac that every family, even the poorest, guarded it jealously," Girolamo Dian wrote in the last century. It was considered an "infallible drug for preserving against the perils of a thousand afflictions that surround humanity."[20]

The prestige of theriac reached its loftiest heights in the seventeenth century; its preparation became the concern of governments, an occasion for a lavish civil and religious ceremony. In Bologna, theriac was prepared with great pomp in the courtyard of the main gymnasium, festively decked out for the occasion. Beneath the curious gazes of an elegant audience, who loudly conversed in the open gallery above, a vast assembly of physicians and apothecaries, aided by servants dressed in green habits with gold epaulettes, mixed the rare and chosen drugs in large, precious vases of majolica.

In Florence, the statute of the apothecaries required that the manufacture of theriac take place in public before selected physicians; a compensation was stipulated for anyone who denounced a suspected adulteration. The *Florentine Prescription Book* mentions that the remedy prepared by the apothecaries was protected from fraud, and cheap theriac, like that imported from Genoa, was seized and burned. Genoa produced such a large quantity that in 1940, the historian Benedicenti found an enormous vase of marble in an ancient pharmacy that still contained a dried residue.[21]

Venice had the highest reputation for quality and refinement. The Serene Republic was favored by the fact that galleys returning from the Orient brought precious and rare drugs. The esteemed pharmacologist Domenico Auda indirectly favored Venice by declaring, with his undisputed authority, that viper flesh did not destroy the poison but only attracted it; the exotic drugs that composed the remedy were responsible for rendering the poison innocuous.

Browsing through the prescriptions of the time, it will be noticed that viper flesh made up only about one-third of the recipe; the rest was composed of an infinity of vegetable substances of common usage added to exotic and rare drugs. Normally, more than sixty ingredients were necessary to prepare the huge mixture, but the experts in each city modified the composition continuously, hoping to excel over the others. Camphor was introduced in Bologna, myrobalan in Rome, swallow-wort, bay, imperatorin, or master-wort in other cities. The ingredients could be increased or changed, providing occasion for fierce and incessant diatribes amongst the learned.

An endless controversy occurred when the redoubtable naturalist, Ulisse Aldrovandi, presumptuously added two rare substances to the Bolognese theriac without waiting for the opinion of the guild of physicians and apothecaries. Aldrovandi won the heated discussion, but the pope in person, supported by two cardinals and the grand duke of Tuscany, was forced to intervene.

More than a hundred substances, necessary for the preparation of "celestial theriac," are listed on a seventeenth-century engraving; the mammoth drug was made with essence of roses, root of gentian, anise seed, cinnamon, scilla, rhubarb, rosemary, pepper, and rare and little-known drugs such as the root of pontentilla Zenziberis, sagapenum, centaury from Asia Minor, galbanum, Cyprus terebinth, Cretian fraxinella, scabious, sandarac, and opobalsam, a resin of the opoponax tree, a plant that grew only in Egypt and was so precious that it was said to be guarded day and night by armed sentries. Since most of the ingredients had a bitter taste, a large quantity of honey was also added.

The archiater of the Duke of Urbino suggested that the heart and liver of deer, wild boars, eagles, vultures, crows or any bird of prey should be added to make the action of the viper flesh more effective. The eminent doctor advised swallowing some of the mighty drug as preventative before a dubious repast in which the guests risked being poisoned by "perfidis hominibus," for it "restored" the temperature of the heart, the liver and the stomach.[22]

Magnificent Preparation Ceremonies

In the sixteenth century, the preparation of theriac in Venice became a festive public event which followed a rigid protocol. The drugs, preserved in precious silver basins, were exhibited "with great pomp and neatly arranged" for at least three days in front of the pharmacy that was to manufacture the drug. In this manner they could be directly inspected by the experts and at the same time displayed to the admiration of all the passersby, whether locals or foreigners. The ingredients were kept in safes, like a treasure, carefully protected against attempts at theft or adulteration by charlatans; the keys were entrusted to the prior of the apothecaries and the treasurer of the magistracy of health. Before the weighing ceremony, "the Chief, Underchief and porters of the pharmacy were each given a black silk cap; that of the Chief was adorned with three plumes, two red and one black; that of the Underchief with two plumes, one red and one black, and that of the porters with one red plume each." The porters who pounded the ingredients in a mortar were offered "a cap of yellow wool with red braid and a red plume," and the porters of the pharmacy, who weighed the substances, were presented with "refreshments of water and lemon, chocolate, and a piece of cake." A small bouquet of flowers with fragrant pieces of cinnamon, placed on a silver tray, was presented to His Excellency the Treasurer and each guest of rank.[23]

In the days that followed, those who were appointed to break up and pound the drugs were recompensed with a generous snack, consisting of "a slice of salami, a slice of cheese, a piece of bread, and a glass of wine." At the end of the lengthy preparation, the theriac was placed in special jars that would be reopened in the presence of the guild of apothecaries after a minimum of two months: A certain period of ripening was considered necessary to allow the mixture to develop all of its curative powers.

The pharmacies that produced theriac were called "theriacal" apothecaries; these shops exhibited signs with their famous names: Testa d'Oro (The Golden Head), Pomo d'Argento (The Silver Apple), l'Aquila Nera (The Black Eagle), the Doge, the Two Moors, and Dello Struzzo (The Ostrich). During the period of preparation, this last pharmacy, which was near the Bridge of the Barettieri, hoisted a large azure banner with the emblem of St. Mark, bearing the written authorization, in "huge golden letters," to manufacture the celebrated remedy.[24]

The magnificence and the solemnity of the Venetian ceremonies was such that at the end of the eighteenth century the extraordinary expenses for the preparation of the drug surpassed the cost of the ingredients. Theriac was produced by now at an industrial pace and was anything but a negligible source of revenue for the Venetian republic, its principle exporter. With a flair for perspicacious publicity, the Venetians claimed that the vipers from the nearby Euganeian hills were particularly suited to the mixture; when an English ambassador questioned this claim, it almost caused a diplomatic incident. As the reptiles became scarce from continuous hunting, they were secretly imported from nearby Slavic regions.

The pharmacies sold many "theriacal" compositions for those who could not afford to buy the valuable drug: The less wealthy could buy "viperine cords," pieces of red cloth with the form and length of a snake, soaked in viper blood and dried, to be applied on ailing parts. These cords were considered particularly valid against inflammations, arthritis, and sore throat.

Viper flesh was regularly entered in official European pharmacopoeia until 1880; many of our great-grandparents may have diligently used it.

In the early nineteen hundreds, theriac was still produced, although without solemnity or the direction of authorities, at the ancient Venetian pharmacy "Testa D'Oro."[25] When the ritual was abandoned in the last century and the first chemical drugs became available, the glorious medicament slowly disappeared, leaving only the elegant, decorated vases that had contained it in the apothecary shops to preserve its memory.

Theriac Imitated

The incredible history of theriac demonstrates that a completely ineffective remedy can have a mysterious therapeutic effect and sometimes stimulate the desired result, but only if the mystical aura that surrounds it and the ritual of its presentation are consonant with the desires of the public and the conviction of physicians. We will never know if a suspicion ever arose in the minds of many eminent doctors and skilled pharmacists that theriac was only a monumental mystification. Francesco Redi must have had some realization when he wrote that many of the doctors' prescriptions, "so beautiful, long, copious, and confused … so nauseous that they would be troublesome for a stomach of marble or iron," are supposed to provoke "so many different effects in so many different parts of our body that they would have to have a hundred hands and a hundred feet and better judgment than the brains of seventy thousand Christians."[26]

The proof that theriac was nothing but an immense deception was indirectly offered by the very people for whom swindling was a trade: the charlatans. The quack Falloppio, not to be confused with the celebrated anatomist of the same name, told how the Bishop of Padua, "in the presence of the Pope, wanted to find out what is most appropriate against poison, and had two chickens poisoned; one was given Theriac, and the other some grass that is called tunic, and the chicken who had taken tunic recovered faster than the one who had theriac."[27] But nothing could change the opinion of the most accredited physicians. Only at the end of the seventeenth century did Don Silvio Boccone, a monk of the Cistercian order, "a studious man who teaches new and beautiful experiences with attention and sincerity," decide that theriac, like mithridate and orvietan, was useful as an antidote for poison only because it provoked vomiting; he pointed out the charlatans who poisoned themselves during their exhibitions and, to induce vomiting, used empirical methods that were more practical, less expensive and above all more efficient than theriac.[28]

Charlatans, attracted by the uncontested success, the glorious reputation and the enormous cost of theriac, decided to make a false one. With their usual shrewdness, they grasped the fact that the complicated remedy did not actually possess any reliable therapeutic effect. Soon they prepared a clever imitation: To achieve more relief from pain, they mixed a little "thebaic" opium into the juices of herbs; to imitate the black color and sweetish taste of theriac, they added a hefty dose of molasses, which was cheaper than honey. The counterfeits made with this healthy sweetener were so successful that some real theriacs were confused with the fake ones and even called "molasses" by the public, causing the irate protests of physicians and apothecaries.

Some impertinent charlatans added salts of antimony to the false theriac, which provoked vomiting; it was an obvious confirmation that the drug had such a vigorous "antipathy" toward poison that it expelled it immediately.

Orvietan: The Charlatans' Sublime Forgery

If orthodox medicine had discovered a powerful remedy of great renown, the charlatans succeeded in making an equally triumphant panacea that was invented from scratch. Orvietan, without a doubt the most successful pharmacological creation of Italian quackery, appeared on the scene at the beginning of the sixteenth century. Sagacious advertising contributed to its attraction and added to the mystery of its jealously guarded, secret composition. Molière, in his "Amour Médicin," sarcastically celebrates the fortune of this remedy:

> Mon remède guérit par sa rare excellence
> Plus de maux qu'on ne peut nombrer dans un an:
> La gale, la rogne, la fievre, la peste, la goutte
> Verole, descente, rougeole…
> O grande puissance de l'Orvietan![29]

> My remedy heals through its rare excellence
> More diseases than can be named in a year:
> Scabies, mange, fever, plague, and gout
> Smallpox, exhaustion, measles…
> O the great might of Orvietan!

For a long time, this mysterious remedy's appeal eclipsed even that of theriac. In 1928, Andrea Corsini wrote that orvietan was sold in France for diseases of livestock until the First World War, and he did not rule out that humans still used it as a personal medicine. In France, the expression "Le merchant d'orvietan," was a synonym for vendor of brews and teller

of tall tales.[30] Using their incomparable rhetoric, the charlatans convinced
the public that their mixture possessed an extraordinary curative potency,
exceeding that of theriac; soon its fame surpassed every limit. Orvietan
served not only as an antidote against poison, snakebite and rabid dogs,
but also against every contagious disease. Quacks, with their innate inge-
niousness, took their clue from the irrationality of the official cure, theriac, whose curative strength supposedly depended on the number and
quality of the ingredients of which it was made. The charlatans maintained that orvietan was a mixture composed of an even larger number of
mysterious substances; they created a sensational drug, in which, except
for laxatives, all the rare and precious substances were counterfeits. What
satisfaction these medical illiterates must have felt when they realized that
the effect of their orvietan was equal, if not superior, to the most celebrated
remedy that orthodox medicine had ever produced.

Orvietan took its name from its inventor, Lupi of Orvieto, "circon-
foraneus aut salta in Banco," who traveled around the Roman countryside, a lowly vagabond who wandered from district to district selling his
remedy, until he finally arrived in the faraway provinces of France. As
often happens with remarkable discoveries, the humble inventor remained
poor and little known, while other quacks achieved considerable gain and
success by exploiting his creation.

One of these was Girolamo Ferrante, who declared that he had come
into possession of the secret; so as not to leave any doubts, he personally
took the name "Orvietano." This sly quack acquired such benevolence and
protection from high-ranking Roman prelates, to whom he provided the
drug free of charge, that the powerful chief physician of Rome, on May 8,
1618, published a broadside, conserved in the Vatican archives, proclaiming, "So that the people will not be duped, and to avoid fraud," that only
the electuary of Girolamo Ferrante alias Orvietano is "good and capable
against all kinds of poison."[31]

The remedy also occasioned a ferocious controversy between Louis
XIV's powerful physician, Theophraste Renaudot, who wanted the therapeutic merits of orvietan to be officially recognized, and the academics of
the University of Paris, led by the polemical Patin. These physicians were
opposed to orvietan more because of their hostility toward the king's doctor than from any real intimate conviction. The Parisian academics won
in the end, but by then the public had given their complete trust to the
remedy. An anonymous Benedictine friar dedicated a booklet to Cardinal
Richelieu with the title "Orvietan for the Melancholic." The friar prescribed orvietan, much as a doctor would prescribe a tranquilizer in our
day, as the best remedy for the scheming cardinal's tired and stressed brain.

At this point it is logical to ask how these two exalted drugs were able to acquire such universal fame and how they could have lasted for such a long time, deceiving entire generations, not only of poor, ignorant peasants, but also of cultured and intelligent people. It is difficult to comprehend how physicians, for hundreds of years, could have maintained their reputations intact, prescribing remedies that were utterly useless, trusting that they would drive out the "peccant" humors just as we now turn to antibiotics to defeat microbes. Even more incomprehensible is the fact that remedies with no biological action could actually produce a curative effect in so many people, as unquestionable as it is mysterious. When we examine these therapeutical eccentricities in a modern and rational light, we must ask how humanity, already decimated by pestilential epidemics, obscure diseases, famine, lack of hygiene and interminable wars could have survived until our day.

The ostentatious rituals used for the preparation of theriac, the words that the charlatans yelled when selling orvietan, were impressed on the public's mind and often ensured the success of the remedy. The elaborate presentation was an irresistible propaganda that provoked an emotional response in each of the onlookers, convincing them that the remedy was unique, extraordinary, magic, exotic, a rare gift. The charlatans often added laxatives to their remedies to prove the swiftness of its effect, a tangible demonstration that it was "working." Nicolò Serpetro recognized this when he wrote that "Guglielmo Parisino had a friend, who without seeing, or touching, or tasting the medicine, but only taking its likeness with his imagination, purged himself."[32]

"Marvelous Secrets"

Medicine and quackery were again twined together in numerous small volumes that revealed many "marvelous secrets." A charlatan of unknown identity took advantage of the celebrated anatomist Gabriele Falloppio's prestige, and, after the academic's death, printed a book of secrets under his name with the pretentious title "Divers and miraculous secrets approved by Physicians of great Fame." The introduction reads: "Who could be so rude and of such an uncouth nature, that he would not enjoy, or even give supreme praise to this useful labor?"[33] The work of the false Falloppio appeared simultaneously with other booklets, was printed in numerous editions in Venice between the sixteenth and seventeenth centuries, then translated and sold in many European countries. There were more than seventy of these books, which treated various subjects of folkloristic medicine. They were so popular that even some licensed physicians, supported by the prominence of their names, were prompted to write on futile topics, until in the end, the number of books written by charlatans was greatly inferior to those written by naturalists and doctors. The authors, because of the subjects they discussed, probably gained more money than any lasting fame.

In reality, these "marvelous secrets," once revealed, were more secret in name than in substance. Usually they were fanciful advice for obtaining health, youth, and beauty, or suggestions that had been gathered from peasants, old women and medicasters of all types. There were instructions on how to make remedies that would conquer diseases and the passage of time, or eliminate the signs of old age and ugliness. Together, physicians and charlatans satisfied the widespread craving to know every arcanum. The public was attracted by nature and preferred the simple advice of empirics to abstract magic, astrological predictions and the vague promises of alchemists.

Following the literary custom of the day, the secrets were preceded by emphatic prologues full of abstruse words; however, on reading, they turned out to be simple and modest suggestions on how to prepare inexpensive remedies without having to depend on the complicated and costly compounds of apothecaries and aromataries. Together with all kinds of medicinal recipes and advice on cosmetics, they often contained directions for organizing conjuring tricks and practical jokes to play on friends. By dealing with the same subjects, doctors and charlatans placed themselves on the same level; both ironically challenged official therapeutics; they were identical cheats, creators of utopia, distributors of amusing and silly fantasies useful only as food for the imagination.

Falloppio suggests: "If you want to change the color of a black horse, take hen droppings and put them on its forehead or another place, and tie it for the night, and in the morning you will find its head white." Pretending modesty, he claims that he does not want to overdo praise of his secrets, so as not to appear like a common quack, "who wants his own remedy to be good for healing all serious infirmities."[34]

At the beginning of the sixteenth century, two charlatans, devout disciples of Giovanni Battista Zapata, "excellent physicians in the Arts and Medicine," printed a book of "Marvelous Secrets of Medicine and Surgery" in honor of their teacher. They tell how to procure remedies within anyone's financial reach: The elderly, the poor, widows and orphans can treat themselves with little cost. Instead of the powdered gems ordered by physicians, prepared with "fine beaten gold, pearls, oriental garnets, hyacinths, rubies, sapphires, emeralds and topaz" that cost "tens of ducats" and are surely not good for "sick stomachs deprived of natural heat," these modest but useful remedies cost only a few coins. There is even advice on how to make a depilatory out of pine resin, wax and turpentine for "anyone who has a hairy face and looks almost like a wild woman."[35]

Medical secrets regarding virility are full of subtle humor and keen good sense. Falloppio prescribes a potion of betony and milk "that makes lust continue, so that if you drink it often, you will be vigorous in that deed." A prosthesis for the penis can be made by catching a large male fox, and then cutting off "the top of his staff, wrapping it in deer skin ... then tie it to your own, and as long as it stays there, his staff will stand up, and will not desert you until you untie it."[36]

An erudite physicist, Pietro Bairo of Turin, physician to Charles II, wrote a compendium of secrets that were useful for "the passions of the staff," but the doctor's advice is even more abstruse than the charlatans'. To "lust," he advises "holding some pieces of a wolf's staff that has been dried in the oven in the mouth" or "powdered bull's staff soaked in fresh egg; all things that will prick it up." For miraculous results, "grease the staff" with oil of mustard or pepper and honey. Another magical secret consists of "rubbing the big toe of the right foot with oil in which blister-beetles have died: it works perfectly." Since the powder of these insects is extremely irritating, "when you want to stop, wash your toe." These and other extravagant ideas, advice not of a charlatan, but of an esteemed physician, are included in a booklet of portable therapy, titled "Vade Meco"; they "serve for all the diseases that can come to Man, starting from the hair of the head down to the soles of the feet."[37]

Under the pseudonym of Reverend Don Alessio Piemontese, the author and naturalist Girolamo Ruscelli wrote a book of "New Secrets." His secret for treating a person "gone out of his mind because of a hex or other reason" is a little startling: After two days of enemas, the patient must be made to swallow a mixture of polypody, or ferns, "and if he doesn't want to take it, tie him up and hold him down by force, opening his mouth and propping it wide with a piece of wood, then throw in the said medicine like one does with horses ... and without doubt, by the grace of God, he will get well."[38]

A skeptical Thomaso Garzoni expressed his own shrewd opinion regarding these successful authors of "secrets": "[T]he secrets of the superstitious are like those of ancient magicians who prescribed, for the cure of quartan fever, to tie cat feces to an owl's toe for seven days" or declared that "the hair of a hyena brought to the lips of a woman has the quality of making her love someone," or that "eating hare for nine continuous days makes a man handsome." These secrets can be useful either as medicines for the body or for the soul, or for beauty alone, or to make money or to show off one's learning, but in order to make these secrets work, "an expert intellect that is trained in profound and obscure matters" is required, someone who knows how to use the powers of suggestion. Unfortunately, most of these medical and quack secretists are "fathers of falsehoods, liars like the Alchemists and Distillers who promise things from the other side of the mountains"; he cautions his readers: "Do not let yourselves be so easily fooled, for more smoke than victuals comes out of the shops of secretists."[39]

CHAPTER 8

"They make robbery seem a courtesy": Italian Charlatans Abroad

The Traveling Aesculapians

At the beginning of the Renaissance, growing numbers of Italian charlatans decided to try their luck beyond the confines of their own country. Encouraged by tales of fabulous profits waiting to be made, they found foreign lands an irresistible temptation. They realized that they would have to overcome the unknown perils of long voyages, the difficulties of new and strange languages, the wariness of authorities suspicious of foreigners, and not least, the hostility of medical colleges and the jealousy of local charlatans. But at the same time, it would be easier for them to seduce a gullible and less wary public, eager to encounter these unconventional personages who dressed with incomparable elegance, talked irresistibly and came with exotic secrets from afar.

Attired in rakish hats and sumptuous velvets embroidered with gold braid, they prepared their monologues with care, cramming their speeches with contorted medical notions, ingenious anecdotes and tales of prodigies. They aimed to stupefy, impress, convince their listeners that before them stood one of "the most excellent doctors in the world," honored and privileged by foreign princes and royalty. They conformed their behavior to please the authorities that would judge them, presenting themselves with austere professional and doctrinal demeanor; when necessary, they did not hesitate to recite grotesque and sarcastic parodies in the style of comedians, often using an improvised interpreter.

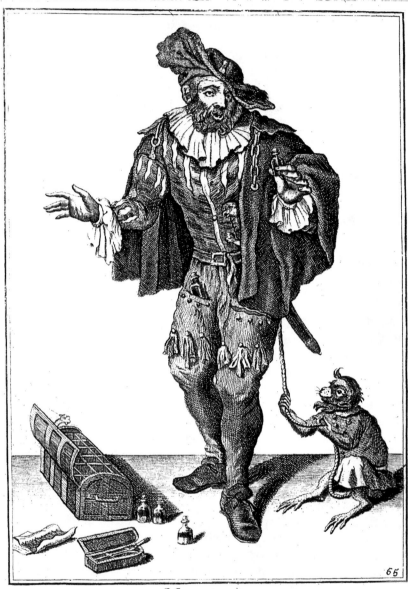

Mountabanck
Le Charlatan
il Ciarlatane

M. auron delin: P. Tempe
                                                                  Excu

An English charlatan dressed in the manner of the Italian quacks. M. Laroon (c.
1700). The Wellcome Institute for the History of Medicine, London.

To remote and little known countries they carried their electuaries, julebs, false theriacs, counterfeit amulets and universal panaceas with pompous names that were supposed to ensure the most absurd cures. Their antidotes for poison were accorded particular favor, as they had been invented in a country like Italy, where poisonings were frequent. Their fraud was presented with panache, so well disguised and with such a refined style that they made "robbery seem a courtesy."[1] On the other hand, honest men were indistinguishable from liars in every country: After his trips through Europe in the sixteenth century, the Florentine ambassador Francesco Vettori commented, "And in effect, the whole world is quackery. Even amongst the erudite, fraud and deceit are the first virtues … and this begins with friars, and goes on amongst magistrates, and physicians, and astrologers, and secular princes…." Vettori confessed an unbounded admiration for those who were able "to find a new art of swindling,"[2] where a cleverly constructed imposture became a triumph of guile. In a world full of duplicity, the Italian quacks quickly intrigued the crowds all over Europe with their talent and their keen, subtle imagination.

Charlatans in England

On a sunny spring day, a great congregation gathered around a platform erected in front of the notorious Tower of London. An elegant quack, who presented himself with the Italian name of Alessandro Bindo, "Honorificicabilitudinitalianibusque doctor," began to harangue the public from the height of his stage, glorifying the qualities of his "Balsam of Balsams": "excellent, hypnotic, captical, odoriferous, carminative, renovative, stiptical, corroboratory" … prepared with moss from a dead man, essence of roses and goose fat — an indispensable remedy for headache, toothache, paralytical paroxysms, rheumatism, gout, fever, fractures and sprains and all the "internal or external miseries, curable or incurable, that strike the human body. The only balsam that holds the true pharmaceutical 'Energy,' prepared by me with art superior to any other medicine that exists in the whole world!"

This bombastic, rambling speech, declaimed in perfect and precise English, did not pour forth from the mouth of an Italian quack, but from that of a well-known English personality: John Wilmot, marquis of Rochester, gentleman of the bedchamber and intimate friend of King Charles II, a nobleman who lived in the middle of the seventeenth century, a wit and poet of lofty lineage who proclaimed himself famous, not only in Europe, but in the Indies, in Africa, and in the Americas; a passionate creator and vendor of remedies against every ailment, and cosmetics that could provide everlasting beauty.[3]

When he mounted his stage for public exhibitions, Wilmot preferred to use an Italian name: Italian quacks were in fact the most convincing orators and the most adept at dealing with the public. Expert connoisseurs of the art of quackery, they repeated in the squares of foreign cities the shows that were typical of Italy. By inventing amusing recitals, employing singers, or harlequins in the guise of servants, or acrobats who danced on a tightrope, they attracted the crowds and convinced them to buy their wares. The exhibition was usually preceded by a display of their false doctoral titles and the presentation of numerous rewards that they had received in all the courts of Europe and the Orient. They peppered their resounding dialogues with incomprehensible phrases in Latin copied from the parlance of physicians or religious ceremonies in their own country.

The English public, hungry for novelties and miracles, was distrustful of the cures of orthodox medicine, and not without reason. The "Gentleman's Magazine" printed letters that recommended the cures of this or that charlatan; various panaceas, along with their price, were listed in the same publication.[4] People of all social conditions chose their healers more for their charisma and capacity to convince than for their official titles. Their longing to discover a portentous remedy encouraged encounters with strange visitors from another land.

When Charles II was crowned king, a particularly favorable era began for Italian charlatans. His benevolence toward these quacks can perhaps be explained by the fact that Italian blood flowed in his veins, inherited from his grandmother, Maria dei Medici. The sovereign was open to the most arcane innovations, anxious to discover new medical utopias, ready to accept and experiment with any remedy. He reinstated on a grand scale the regal "touch" with which he cured the scrofulous and generously conferred licenses to foreign quacks, overcoming with his higher authority the jealous resistance of the medical colleges. Any foreign charlatan who applied for a license was required to pay roughly a hundred pounds, an inaccessible sum for an itinerant salesmen, but often they were able to acquire a permit thanks to the protection of a person who was influential at court or the backing of an illustrious personality who had been seduced by the gift of a "pharmaceutical sample," a remedy brought from Italy — a bold attempt on the part of the charlatan to acquire patronage, linked to the result of the miraculous specific. If fortune were benign, if the force of suggestion worked its magic and the cure achieved the desired result, sponsorship and a license were assured. With luck, fame and fortune would follow.

L.G. Matthews collected some of the scarce and often incomplete information about those quacks who came to England from regions all over Italy. A Sicilian, Salvatore Mosca, solemnly promised to cure those who were blind from birth, free of charge. His dialogue was so persuasive that the poor wretches were convinced that they had seen an illusory, tenuous ray of light.[5] Another Italian charlatan, Micha (Michele) Philo, obtained a temporary license and was so adroit that the king rewarded him with an order to the authorities: "Give the Italian every due reception, and (do) not permit that other charlatans dare mount their platforms close to his, or molest him in any way."[6]

Not all foreign quacks had the same good fortune: Bartolomeo Silva from Turin was found ignorant in medicine and philosophy, refused a license, fined and put in prison. However, this case was fairly rare, for generally the authorities failed to realize, or pretended not to notice, that many of these Italian "doctors" did not even know how to read and write.[7]

The "Elixir Vitae, which keeps fatigue away and lengthens life," was successfully presented by Salvatore Winter, a quick-witted Neapolitan, whose real name was Inverno; it was sufficient to smell his specific or at the most take a few spoonfuls a day to "resuscitate a great number of persons who should have died." The offer of his celebrated Elixir was preceded by a brief but moving ceremony in which the charlatan offered thanks to almighty God.

In 1608 Filippo Bernardini peddled Archicatharticum in London, a remedy that was wrapped in paper printed with Gregorian chants; the charlatan, who probably offended the touchy and ferociously antipapist English clergy, ended up in jail until he was able to pay a fine. Although the zealous protestant ministers invoked the stake for these Catholic quacks, no Italian was actually ever burned. Some English quacks even seemed to feel a certain nostalgia for the Catholic church, for they offered "Vatican pills" for sale, or false relics of saints, or the famous "pulvis benedictius" that had more success as a miracle than as a medicine.[8] In 1700, William Patence, dentist to the royal family, presented his "universal medicine" with the name "Catholicon," a panacea that cured most known diseases and carried a guarantee of reimbursement if the remedy failed to work.[9] The origin of the name probably came from a legend which recounted how angels brought the divine remedy Catholicon to Charlemagne, as preventive against a terrible epidemic of plague.

Locatelli, a shrewd quack from Genoa, introduced his electuary with the name, "Italian Balsam," a mixture that became so renowned that later it could be found in the *London Pharmaceutical* list of drugs. It was a mixture that anticipated the Mediterranean diet by four centuries: olive oil and red Italian wine figured amongst its ingredients, along with "dragon's blood" made from red sandalwood.

An enterprising Sicilian, Pasqua Rose, opened the first "coffee house" in London, introducing the aromatic drink. In perfect charlatanesque style, he extolled the therapeutic virtues of coffee in a printed handbill. Another Italian, with the Latin-sounding name of Giovanni Puntaeus,[10] was embroiled in a violent dispute. While Puntaeus was selling his orvietan and vaunting its miraculous effects against poison, an English doctor, jealous of his success, denied his claims. The argument ended, as can be easily imagined, with an experiment on the Italian charlatan's servant. A dose of "aqua fortis," a strong poison, was given to the brave man who, well trained in the trick, pretended to swallow it and expire. He revived the next day, obviously after a dose of orvietan dispensed by his master.

Charlatans in Spain and France

Unlawful medical practice had spread like a scourge through Europe for many years. In the early fourteenth century, Philip the Fair's chief surgeon, Henry de Monville, made a report on the enormous number of false physicians who sold remedies of every kind: Amongst these, along with common charlatans, were spurious barbers, chiromancers, counterfeiters, midwives, old women, and even some clerics and nobles, but the worst of all were converted Jews and Saracens, for de Monville suspected the latter of spying secrets from the state for the purpose of revealing them to the enemy.

In fifteenth-century Spain, many people preferred the celebrated "moriscos," the heirs of Arab popular medicine. These sorcerers and magicians held great prestige, not only amongst the common folk but also within the dominant Catholic hierarchy, the rich bourgeoisie, and the royal court. They normally stepped in only when the physician had left the patient in God's hands. In the sixteenth century, academic medicine's opposition became stronger, and the Holy Inquisition accused the moriscos of crimes against Christianity, witchcraft, sodomy, hermaphroditism, and even of alliance with the hated Turks and pirates of Barbary.

Some of these charlatans arrived in Italy. The passage of an empirical herbalist from Valenza, who took the Italian name Giovanni di Giovanni, is noted in a curious fifteenth-century document discovered in the archives of Foligno in Umbria, a demonstration that entertainment and recreation went hand in hand with the sale of remedies. An itinerant Sienese bard, who had been given the Catalonian nickname of "El Zoppo" (the Lame One), was hired for a daily salary of twenty-five "baiocchi," or small silver coins, by di Giovanni, who sold a powder against worms. A bona fide contract in Latin was written up between the two, properly countersigned by respected citizens who acted as witnesses. The bard pledged to sing or tell stories or fables twice a day for a whole year; between one song and the next, the charlatan pursued his business, which must have been profitable enough, if it allowed him to employ a singer.[11]

In France, the most numerous and the most sought-after foreign charlatans were Italians, almost until the end of the eighteenth century. The invasion of Italian quacks was imputed to two Italian queens, Catherine and Maria de' Medici, who were generally disliked. Amongst the many foul deeds attributed to them was the introduction of all sorts of adventurers into France, an unjust accusation, for in the preceding centuries the vicinity of the two countries had favored the arrival of merchants and bankers, followed by wheeler-dealers, schemers, and vagabonds of every kind.

As early as the fourteenth century, an Italian charlatan, Angelo Catto, had become famous at the court of Louis XII. When the monarch had a stroke, Catto, who claimed to be a famous physician, cared for him with judicious skill. Perhaps it was only an episode of transient cerebral ischemia, for the king's health returned in a few days, and the sudden apoplectic stroke transformed itself into a stroke of good luck for the charlatan. Faithful to his motto, "Ingenium superat vires" ("Intelligence overcomes strength"), he took advantage of the providential recovery by awarding all the merit to his own remedies. Catto gratified the king's passion for astrology, leading him to believe that his knowledge of the stars allowed him to foresee the most important events that would occur during the king's reign; actually, he obtained most of the information through his own personal, secret system of swift messengers. After Catto returned to Italy, he boasted that the grateful king, impressed by his divinatory powers, offered him nothing less than the archbishopric of Vienna, which Catto modestly refused.[12]

Giovanni Bissoni from Bologna was amongst the charlatans who moved to France at the end of the eighteenth century; at the age of fifteen he had worked for an elderly quack named Girolamo, a monger of unguents and balsams. The boy served as sidekick for his master, doing his utmost to make people laugh at his ridiculous jokes. Soon the pupil surpassed his teacher and moved on alone with his jars and bottles to Milan. There he found that his ancient master had taken up a place in the square. Refusing to be intimidated, the young quack placed his own platform nearby and began to recount a pathetic tale, confessing that he was the degenerate son of the old man and had come to beg his pardon. The elderly quack became more and more enraged and began to curse the young man. The audience, fooled by the clever young comedian's story, felt such pity for him that to console him, they rushed to buy all his wares. Bissoni continued to travel, sometimes alternating his role as quack doctor with that of comedian in the parts of Scapino or Finocchio, two scheming, sly, and witty stock characters in Italian theater. Bissoni was such a consummate actor that the French audiences who watched his performances cried for him to take off his mask so that could better see "the passions" that illuminated his face.[13]

Quackery in Paris

In comparison with the long, dour, complicated disquisitions of orthodox physicians, Italian charlatans brought merriment, laughter, and fresh hopes to the crowds who thronged around their platforms near the Pont Neuf or Place Dauphine. For their advertising, they used the public criers who were employed in front of churches and at markets to inform the public of royal edicts and judgments of the courts. For a few coins these criers, during their free time, would declaim the infinite curative properties of elixirs, nectars and balsams and the virtues of a host of remedies, from the prodigious theriac to the more domestic chamomile, which young ladies could use to "wash their asses and the rest."

At the Pont Neuf, Melchiorre Barri sold his "Peruvian Pomade," which erased the pustules of small pox, a "Japanese Unguent" that dyed white hair, and a "Chinese Quintessence," which made the eyes bigger and shrank the mouth. He told his listeners how his famous "Universal Unguent" had not only cured the king of legendary Siam, but his white elephant as well, and he moved the crowd with tales of the huge feasts given in his honor by the great mogul and the emperor of Morocco.[14]

Paris had by now become the capital of empirics and charlatans, and amongst these, the Italians were the most numerous and the most admired. Their manner of dressing was adapted to the refined elegance of the larger French cities; in challenges with their local rivals they wore bright-colored clothes, plumed hats and gold chains. They organized their troupe's spectacles with the talent of accomplished comedians. Their stages were always surrounded by crowds, for an Italian name was sufficient to attract an audience.

The Famous Tabarin

One of the most celebrated Parisian charlatans was Tabarin, who lived in the first decades of the seventeenth century. The admired actor and medicine vendor's origins are unknown: Since mystery was an added attraction for the public, he did his utmost to hide his past beneath a veil of secrecy; even so, he sometimes let slip that he had been born in Naples. In his history of Neapolitan theater, Benedetto Croce quotes Fluidoro, an ancient chronicler, who tells of a mountebank called Tabarrino or Tamburrino. This charlatan from Savoy had a company of strolling players whom he paid to recite in Piazza Castello in Naples; since "the concourse is great without paying … he sells a conserve of juniper for antipoison, disposing of a large amount, and he heals scrofula or rather cold abscesses."[15] The quack, "intrinsically most interesting and two faced in behavior and in feature," attracted the crowds with his strange habit of acting and dressing as a Savoyard. He spoke fluent French, and his wife, Vittoria Branca, was certainly of Italian origin.

Tabarin presented his balsams, salves for sores, ointments for burns, and electuaries for toothache on the Isle de la Cité, in front of a huge crowd. As a small orchestra of violas and violins struck up a melody, his wife danced for the audience, who bought the remedies gladly so that they could watch the show. Tabarin would appear on stage, wearing a popular Pierrot costume, a large, modish felt hat perched atop his long white hair; his beard, like the god Neptune's, had three tips, and he held a long wooden sword. The comedy began with the arrival on the scene of Modor, who played the part of an erudite physician-philosopher, dressed in an ample, white linen cape covered with decorations. The public was vastly entertained by the contrast between the two strange characters and their amusing dialogue. At first attentive and silent, they then began to laugh until they cried. Tabarin, a witty and sarcastic jester, asked continuous, extravagant questions that mocked and ridiculed the professor's science, based on theory and difficult words. The public adored Tabarin, for he impersonated one of the common people; he used age-old common shrewdness as a weapon against the vain physician, the haughty pedant who professed the eloquent doctrine of a know-it-all.

It is impossible to know if the famous Tabarin of Paris was in reality that same Tamburrino who performed in the Neapolitan squares, but at the end of his career, Tabarin mysteriously confessed that he was descended from the god Saturn, whose son, born in southern Italy, was named Tabarum; whatever the truth, this celebrated Parisian charlatan's conduct and his manner of presenting himself to the public was typical of an Italian quack.

Gerolamo Ferrante's Success in Paris

In the seventeenth century, the squares of Paris were the setting for the exploits of the master charlatan Gerolamo Ferrante. The acclaimed star of his company was Galinette La Galina, a lovely damsel who sang, accompanied by violas, and amused the audience by reciting risqué pleasantries. What better expedient could there be to attract a crowd and introduce the charlatan's orvietan, the gargantuan remedy that had been invented by Italian quacks?

In France, orvietan surpassed the legendary theriac in the public's fantasy. A pill "the size of a hazelnut" was sufficient to prevent poisoning and cure any type of disease. As soon as they had perceived a good deal, other local quacks improvised themselves as orvietan vendors and made considerable profits by copying Ferrante's act.

The saga of orvietan did not end with Ferrante's death. His wife Clarissa, heir to his property and his secrets, married two more charlatans in succession. She tied the knot first with a French doctor named Vetrier, who was soon convinced that it was more profitable to set up a stage and change his French name to an Italian "Tramontano." When she became a widow once more, Clarissa wed another Italian, Contugi, who qualified himself as "the real heir of the secret of orvietan," and declared to all who would listen that, thanks to his wife, he was the sole possessor of Ferrante's medicinal treatises.

Contugi proved to be a vendor of superior temperament and ingenuity. Still following in the tradition of Italian charlatans, he combined the sale of his remedies with a show, organizing a troupe of comedians and taking for himself the role of Captain Spaccamondo. His success was immediate, and in 1647 he obtained the permission to make and sell orvietan under the seal and benevolent patronage of the Sun King. The original copy of the "privilege" granted to Contugi by the king's chancellor is reproduced in an elegant engraving, decorated with the sovereign's insignia and crest depicting the sun, and framed with a series of drawings: snakes, poisonous mushrooms, scorpions, crabs, tarantulas, toads and salamanders. The document declares that by order of the king, Jean Louis Contugi is the only true owner of the secret of Roman orvietan, and the only heir to Jean Vetrier, who in turn was successor to Gerolamo Ferrante: a recognized royal license for a celebrated dynasty of orvietan charlatans.

The privilege caused fierce protests from the powerful guilds of physicians and apothecaries. In their naive complaint, they demanded to know how Contugi could procure all the necessary drugs for the enormous amount of orvietan that he produced. Contugi's whole life was marked by furious disputes and judicial controversies, but he had to defend himself more from counterfeiters than from the medical hierarchy. He was surrounded by rivals who sold coarse imitations of the drug everywhere and who claimed to have changed the secret of his composition only to make it more potent. A French quack, Regnaud, who had his platform in Rue Dauphine, even had the nerve to sell orvietan right in front of Contugi, copying, Contugi sarcastically remarked, "my watch and my boots."

After Contugi's death, fourteen of his sons inherited the secret and the exclusive license to manufacture orvietan. For most of their lives they lived in the shadow of the Pont Neuf, which had witnessed their celebrated father's feats for so many years. Toward the end of the eighteenth century, the sons sold the recipe for a considerable amount of money, but by that time the licenses for its manufacture in Europe were countless, granted by the authorities to herbalists, botanists, pharmacists, physicians, and even to journalists.[16]

A Tuscan Marquis and Traveling Quack

A history of Italian charlatans who practiced their trade abroad would not be complete without mentioning Nicolò Cevoli del Carretto, the descendant of a noble family of Pisa. In Flanders and later in Paris, his flair for alchemy and the practice of medicine made him rich and famous, but his life was continuously troubled by disputes with French doctors, who could not abide the witty expedients of the noble foreigner who so cleverly exploited his noble title and his glib tongue. Their hatred and envy was increased by the brilliant charlatan's effortless success: They scornfully denounced his writings, filled "with foolishness, with falsehoods and deceits, to trick the populace and idiots." They accused him quite rightly of exhibiting false doctoral titles, but the young marquis answered that he had only lowered himself to practice medicine because of his languishing financial condition, an affirmation so insulting that it further infuriated his detractors.

After making a fortune with his "Tincture of the Moon," an infallible remedy against epilepsy, he began to sell, with popular success and considerable profit, his "Grand Remedy" or "Well Water of the Marquis de Carretto." With unbelievable impudence, he claimed that the remedy was made out of the water from the wells of his own home, and that anyone could buy it directly at his Parisian residence in Rue de la Seine. The water would conserve youth and vigor and delay old age and death, obviously "only until the term prescribed by the Master of Life and Death."[17]

The largest bottle cost an extravagant "hundred pistoles," or gold coins, but to obtain its magical effects one had to take only seven drops a day. The marquise of Sevigné, his devoted friend and a passionate consumer, peremptorily advised her friends to "drink Carretto or Vichy!" By the grace of his noble name and the approval of his high-ranking friendships, the water from his wells had became miraculous.

It was his quarrelsome disposition, and not the profession of charlatan, which finally brought him to ruin. Believing himself the victim of an injustice because he had been denied an inheritance in his own country, he dispatched abusive letters to his enemies and finally even accused the magistrates of corruption. Betrayed by nostalgia for the beautiful Tuscany of his birth, toward the end of the seventeenth century, he left for Italy and was soon afterward arrested by order of Cosimo III de' Medici, who had him locked up in the fortress of Volterra. Feigning sickness, he begged for clemency, but to no avail. He disappeared, like Cagliostro, in some secret dungeon, a destiny common to many unfortunate adventurers of his time.

Hordes of Italian Aesculapians still continued to emigrate to wealthy and powerful France, but the times were changing: Local quacks had taken possession of the lucrative trade in remedies, and the Italians had to deal with Spanish, Polish and German charlatans as well. In an attempt to stem the invasion, French laws became stricter, and to avoid being condemned for illegal practice of medicine, illiterate charlatans often had to hire a French doctor to sign their prescriptions. Although laws were unable to stop them, the shadow of the French Revolution finally caused them to disappear for a time.

"Divine Borri" and His Celestial Mission

Late at night on the 13th of August, 1695, a cart reserved for the transport of the dead collected the body of Francesco Giuseppe Borri from the dungeons of Castel Sant'Angelo in Rome and took it to the Church of S. Maria in Traspontina. There it was given a Christian burial, the sole concession that the pope, Innocent XII, had allowed to the heretic that he had persecuted, captured and condemned to the stake, a sentence that only later had been commuted to life in prison. Thus the most important charlatan doctor of the seventeenth century disappeared in gloomy silence, like an unknown swindler.

During his life, Giuseppe Francesco Borri had distinguished himself as an extraordinary healer and an ambitious philosopher and alchemist.

He spent his earthly existence searching obsessively for the Philosopher's Stone, that ultimate fount of knowledge and prosperity, the source of all physical and mental health. To fulfill this quest, he practiced a medicine that was based on chemical experiments and hermetic theories. His success as a doctor was contrasted by the contempt, intolerance and condemnation of the ecclesiastics, who could not forgive his rebellious ideas and restless spirit.

Young Giuseppe Francesco Borri had been born under a lucky star: Son of a well-known Milanese doctor and amateur alchemist, he was privileged enough to be accepted, at the age of sixteen, into a strict Jesuit seminary in Rome, a school which offered an exclusive education and had been attended by future cardinals and popes. The rector who welcomed the elegant young man could certainly not have foreseen the turbulence that this pupil was to bring to the austere religious institution. Although he was recognized by his teachers as "a young man of marvelous intellect and prodigious memory," Borri soon revealed his undisciplined temperament; his spirit was so rebellious that he organized other pupils into a revolt; the governor's bailiffs had to be called in, and Borri was expelled from the seminary.

Despite the splendor of its new churches, fountains and palaces, Rome was a turbulent city in the seventeenth century. Corrupted by the pope's odious nepotism, it was torn asunder by riots and anarchy, by struggles between rival bands and continuous brawls and duels. In this atmosphere, after a period of youthful dissoluteness, forever in rebellion against the society in which he lived, Borri began to expound his strange ideas. Following in his father's footsteps, he had dedicated himself to the study of alchemy ever since the days when he was a boarder at the Jesuit school. A fervent critic of Galenic medicine, he had occasionally attended the medical school of the university "La Sapienza" before beginning his own practice as a healer. His weird remedies, which he composed himself, soon earned him his first successes, not only with the poor, but with wealthy patricians as well. His flattering and convincing words and attractive appearance made him the darling of Roman society. Amongst his many illustrious friends was Christina of Sweden, the eccentric queen whose desire to "make gold" would become one of the causes of Borri's misfortunes. His fate changed abruptly when he began to meddle in religious issues, "turning against God," as the Dominican judges pronounced in the trial that was brought against him, "the talent that had been benignly bestowed upon him."

Seized by a mystical vision, in revolt against the political and religious situation of the times, Borri boldly dreamed of a new world, one and united, made peaceful by the conversion of all nations; this would be accomplished militarily under the intangible guidance of the pope. Borri revealed to his numerous followers that the Archangel Michael had personally given him a sword engraved with the signs of the seven truths; whoever dared oppose him would be destroyed by the celestial armies, of which Borri would soon become the captain general. Borri nonchalantly declared that he was on familiar terms with the Sublime Seraphims and the Joyful Angels, to whose benevolence he owed his marvelous gifts of healing. Wounded in a duel, he swore that he had been saved from certain death by intercession of the Virgin Mary, who had appeared to him in a heavenly vision, a vision so indelible that he would later insist that the Holy Eucharist contained a particle of the Mother of God. Borri had gone beyond every limit, and the Inquisition was left without doubt: The heretical theories of the rebellious youth were unforgivable and deserving of punishment. To Borri's misfortune, Alexander VII had recently ascended the papal throne, firmly convinced that stringent rules should be imposed against any religious deviance.

While the Holy Inquisition, instigated by the powerful Cardinal Pignatelli, "deprived him of every honor and prerogative" and condemned him to death on the stake, Borri, declaring himself ready for his celestial mission, gathered numerous proselytes. By the time the order for his arrest arrived, he was already in Milan, driven more by the epidemic of plague that at that time was raging through Rome than by any fear of being arrested. Disregarding the sentence, he continued unperturbed for another four years, propagandizing his heresies and gathering disciples in the city of his birth. The tribunal of the Holy Inquisition finally ordered that he be apprehended and transferred to Rome in chains. Borri made a fortuitous escape: While his followers were being arrested, he was already far away, taking refuge in Switzerland, where he was certain of protection. Condemned in absentia to death by burning, his image, "painted from life, … was carried on a wagon through Rome to the sound of trumpets, so that the people would run to see it, and then after being hanged, it was burned in Campo dei Fiori." But Borri was still free, and it was said that with his usual impudence he had declared, after the ceremony of the "burning," that he had never felt as cold as he had at that hour, on that day.[18]

A Papal Prison and a Guardian Angel

Borri began a new life, traveling to various European capitals. After Switzerland, he went to Innsbruck and Strasbourg, always preceded by his fame as an excellent physician and prodigious alchemist.

Once in Amsterdam, at that time one of the richest and most important cities in Europe, the imaginative refugee abandoned his dangerous heretical ideas once and for all and consolidated his fortune as a healer. In the homeland of Protestantism, Borri was also able to don the halo of a martyr of the Inquisition.

Soon, the renown of his healings spread through Europe; crowds of patients waited in his antechambers to receive his miraculous secrets. He visited the poor without charge; some came on litters from nearby countries to be cured by the man who justly deserved the title of "universal physician." All were won over by his extraordinary healings, and he was called "doctor of miracles." Inebriated by his easy success, Borri assumed the title of "excellency" and installed himself in one of the most sumptuous residences in the city.[19] Surrounded by a numerous court of servants dressed in elegant liveries, he began a luxurious and expensive lifestyle. It is a mystery how this fugitive was able to spend such enormous sums, especially since he had been deprived, by order of the Inquisition, of his paternal inheritance. A great part of his ostentatious wealth was the fruit of ingenious chemical tricks: He fabricated and sold false pearls, but above all he deceived those who waited trustfully for his promised transmutation of base metals into gold. Like other successful adventurers, it is conceivable that he possessed, along with his undeniable charisma, hypnotical powers which emanated from "his green eyes, like two stars out of which shined a Spirit almost superior to the Human."[20]

The figure of the benevolent physician contrasted with the soul of the mystifier; he continued his alchemical research with passion, spreading the word that the discovery of the Philosopher's Stone was imminent. The news reached the English medical establishment, and a group of eminent physicians came seeking an explanation. Borri returned their admiration with sibylline answers, and the doctors returned home without the stone, content with his gift of a new secret against the plague.

Soon the expenditures for his experiments in alchemy and his exalted standard of living became untenable, and he was obliged to dismiss his servants in livery and put his sumptuous carriages and purebred horses up for sale. When he realized that his reputation was beginning to tarnish and that criticisms and suspicions were beginning to be aired, he decided that it was time to move on.

He moved his residence to Hamburg, where he attempted to change metals into gold for his friend, Queen Christina of Sweden, but soon he abandoned her court and moved to Denmark. King Frederick III, in spite of the rumors of Borri's frauds, gave him a warm welcome and provided him with magnificent new equipment for his alchemical experiments.

Borri could now renew his research, continuously urged on by the impatient monarch, who hoped that the gold which would come out of the charlatan's "philosophical furnace" would enable him to buy Peru! Unfortunately, although the famous alchemist and his helpers labored feverishly over alembics and crucibles, the noble metal refused to appear. Each time, Borri's continuous, self-assured excuses persuaded the sovereign that the accusations of quackery were unfounded; with canny intuition, Borri offered medical advice and even highly appreciated political opinions.

With the death of King Frederick, Borri's security began to vacillate. His luck was beginning to run out, and perhaps in a case of mistaken identity, he was arrested and taken to Vienna. Cardinal Pignatelli, who had ordered his arrest years before, had recently arrived in Austria as the Apostolic Nuntius. Despite the protection of the emperor, the high-ranking prelate succeeded in having Borri extradited and escorted to Rome under heavy guard.

At first, he enjoyed some freedom in the city where he had spent the turbulent years of his youth; thanks to his important connections and to his belated repentance, he was able to have his death sentence commuted to life imprisonment. Like every repentant heretic, he was obliged to perform a public abjuration; the ceremony took place in front of the judges of the Inquisition in the church of the Minerva, before a huge and noisy gathering. Egidio de' Magri, a chronicler of the time, describes Borri: "guilty, dressed in the attire of the Inquisition, a tunic of black silk without a collar ... red crosses painted on the breast and on the back, hands and feet bound in chains, kneeling on the scaffold's platform with a candle by his right side," fainting while the crowd outside screams, "Burn him, burn him!" Brought to his senses with vinegar, he was publicly reminded of his heresy; since he had admitted and confessed his error and asked for forgiveness, he was absolved from "greater excommunication" which would have led inexorably to the stake. As "salutary penitence" it was mandated that for the rest of his life he recite every day the "Apostolic Symbol."[21]

In the beginning, his incarceration was light: He had a final stroke of luck when he miraculously cured the powerful French ambassador, Duke Cardinal Destrée, who had fallen seriously ill. It was such an extraordinary event that an ironical lampoon went around the city stating that, "In Rome it takes a heretic to perform miracles." The same voluble populace who a short time before had demanded that he be burned at the stake now sang the praises of the great healer.

But when Cardinal Pignatelli donned the papal tiara with the name of Innocent XII, Borri's imprisonment turned harsh; once again pity was

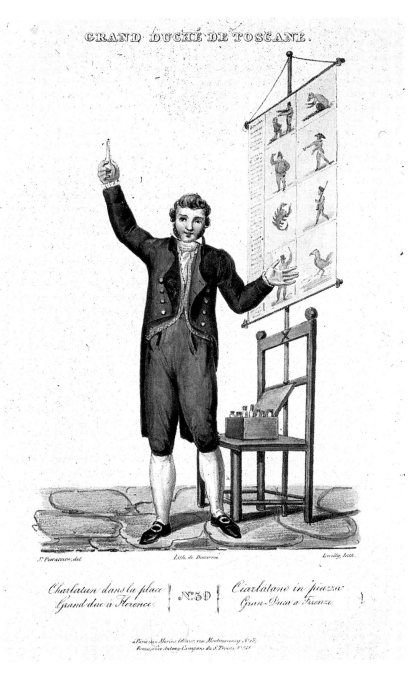

An itinerant vendor offering his products in Florence. F. Pieraccini e Levily, France (c. 1700). Biblioteca Nazionale Centrale, Firenze.

denied him, although it was said that during attacks of gout, the new pope was restored by warm baths of hare's blood, prescribed by the charlatan. Miraculous healing abilities were still attributed to the celebrated adventurer, even as he was locked up, heavy hearted and sick, in the forbidding papal prison; he was so famous that after his death more than seven thousand requests were found in the chambers of Castel Sant'Angelo from citizens of every condition asking permission to visit him in the hope of regaining their lost health.

The "paludum effluviis," or "pernicious fever" of malaria, that infested the countryside and the Roman suburbs had by now inexorably sapped Borri's body; with empirical intuition, during the quaking fevers he asked in vain to try quinine powder, the miraculous "cinchona" which had recently been brought from the far Americas by a Jesuit priest. But the prodigious remedy for malaria, which perhaps would have saved him, never arrived. It seemed as if the same Jesuits who had welcomed him as a student in their seminary when he was a reckless youth still refused to forgive his defiant rebellion.

The most celebrated alchemist and medical charlatan of his time died like a common criminal in the bleak papal prison. During his final, interminable nights, the man who had been known as "Divine Borri" may have turned his thoughts to the statue of the Archangel Michael in the act of sheathing his sword, placed on the highest rampart of the Castel Sant'Angelo as the symbol of the Roman populace's gratitude for having brought the terrible plague to an end. During Borri's last days, the blessed archangel may no longer have appeared to him as the revolutionary head of celestial armies, but as his serene guardian angel.

CHAPTER 9

The Alfier Lombardo, the Unknown Knight, and a Charlatan Doctor

The "Honored Tooth Drawers"

An engraving by Maggiotto depicts a poor wretch as he pleads, "For the love of God, remove my distress... But do not unhinge my jaw!" A bewigged quack, attired in an elegant, eighteenth-century costume, strains in the gargantuan attempt to extract an unyielding tooth from the mouth of a peasant who has almost collapsed at his feet. Many artists have mockingly illustrated the operation of pulling teeth, emphasizing the patient's desperation as he gasps and flails his arms, legs wide apart and thrashing from the unbearable pain.

The art of drawing teeth is invariably coupled with the specter of pain and fear; nowadays, although the former has mostly been done away with, the latter still remains. It is impossible to count the inventions, since ancient times, of novel instruments for pulling teeth or to number the attempts, as various as they were ineffectual, to replace missing teeth with false ones. Elegant Etruscan, Egyptian, and Roman prostheses in gold can be admired in museums, but few of them were able to sustain the wear and tear of use. Horace recounts the story of the old witch Canidi, who, while in a cemetery gathering bones for her macabre sorcery, was frightened by Priapus's thunderous fart; she precipitously fled, dropping her false teeth on the ground during her escape.

Some of the most able tooth drawers were even celebrated by orthodox physicians and became famous for their ability, dexterity, and daring.

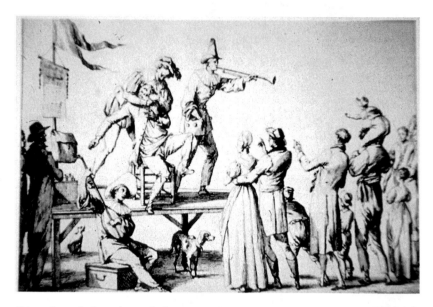

L'Arracheur de dents (A tooth drawer). A clown blows his horn to cover the patient's shrieks. J. Duplessi-Bertaux (1710. U.S. National Library of Medicine, Bethesda, MD.

Unless the teeth to be pulled were wobbly or milk teeth, the art of extraction was a difficult task, an arduous responsibility, an insidious adventure; the outcome was so uncertain that physicians and surgeons willingly left this thankless charge to the despised quacks. The tooth drawer could fail in his attempt to pull a tooth deeply rooted in its socket, and often dangerous and unforeseen consequences such as hemorrhages or infections occurred. For centuries, many quacks made tooth drawing their exclusive specialty — a profession that some vagabonds, both humble and renowned, willingly accepted, aware that a successful extraction could not only earn good money, but assure fame and prestige. The operation was presented to the immediate verdict of the crowd that pressed around the tooth drawer's platform, and this gave them a chance to sell remedies for every sort of affliction. Extractions were often so difficult that some clever tooth drawers, to demonstrate their prowess, pretended to remove the tooth with the tip of their sword while sitting on a gaily caparisoned horse: a spectacular demonstration, worthy of an illusionist. A false tooth was shown round to the public while a helper applied opiate paste to the mouth of the hapless patient, in an attempt to alleviate the pain.

An ingenious inventor, toward the end of the eighteenth century, had the brilliant idea of extracting teeth by means of pliers attached to a pistol. The barrel was inserted into the patient's mouth and with one shot the tooth was extracted and a blank was fired with an earsplitting explosion, inducing anesthesia "from fright"—noisy, but apparently effective.[1]

The extraction of teeth required uncommon energy and strength, and the operator had to master the ability of propping himself on his legs. In a letter to the College of Physicians, the physician of Serra, a small town near Siena, praises a local charlatan, a tooth drawer so expert in assuming "the point of support [that] he has concluded infinite extractions with felicitous success and without causing the least harm."[2]

Pulling teeth in such an energetic manner exposed the jaw to the risk of fracture. "Dentem sì, non maxillam" ("The tooth yes, not the jaw") was inscribed on the banner of Grand Thomas, a renowned "arracheur de dents" who lived during the reign of Louis XV. A man of gigantic stature with a booming voice, Grand Thomas was wildly adored by hordes of admirers. He performed on a platform covered with a roof surmounted with the emblem of a huge, crowned tooth. Like his Italian colleagues, he carried a long sword with which he pretended to draw recalcitrant teeth; before the operation, the patient kneeled before him, and Grand Thomas, endowed with the strength of a bull, lifted him three times off the ground. To honor the birth of the dauphin, Grand Thomas traveled to Versailles dressed in a scarlet, oriental costume decorated with trophies of the teeth he had extracted, wearing a hat of solid silver, sixteen inches high and seven wide. Even his horse's saddle was adorned with teeth strung as beads, one after the other. The legendary hero was preceded by a gonfalon embroidered with drops of blood in enamel and teeth in the guise of stars.[3]

Successful extractions, performed swiftly and dexterously where other unskilled tooth drawers, to their disparagement and shame, had failed, could earn the boundless admiration of any public who witnessed the operation. At the sight of a cured and grateful patient, who only a short time before, with swollen jaw, had been screaming from the unbearable stabs of pain, the enthusiastic crowd transformed a modest tooth drawer into a "professor dentist," a healer who might possess, besides the competence of his hands, the knowledge to cure many other ailments. The triumphant charlatan did not allow these favorable opportunities to escape, for they repaid him for all the efforts and risks of his trade: After a difficult extraction with a fortunate outcome, he could offer his incomparable "secret," a remedy that not only would "heal rotten teeth, consolidate the wobbly, comfort the stupefied (sensitive) and the frigid," but could heal all other afflictions.

In the sixteenth century, even if tooth drawing was considered a social necessity, the fact that these charlatans took advantage of their success to sell forbidden remedies caused the stern Venetian College of Physicians to protest. The doges issued bans prohibiting the sale of remedies, and the penalties were not to be taken lightly: The transgressor could be condemned to be a "man of oars" for eighteen months on a Venetian galley; habitual offenders received six months of "bolted prison" which was followed by five years of exile.[4]

With time, considering the usefulness of tooth drawers and the uselessness of admonitions and penalties, the Colleges of Physicians were obliged to turn a blind eye; an endless series of boastful announcements vaunting the virtues of incomparable remedies for toothache and diseases of the mouth were printed in the gazettes or advertising sheets or inserted in the midst of requests for licenses that can still be found in the medical colleges' collections of correspondence.

The Angelical Vulnerary Elixir that Bortolo Pirazzi sold in 1770 must have possessed illimitable therapeutical properties: The list of substances of which it was composed take up four finely written pages of his manuscript. Spirit of wine, saffron, calamus (sedge), angelica, sandal, and "dragon's blood" were only a few of the drugs used in this composite medicine. Pirazzi recommended that it be kept "under horse manure for twenty-four days or in the sun for forty days." Once the time was up, the charlatan could be certain that the toothache had disappeared.[5]

As a strengthener for loose, or "icy" teeth, there were opiates, preparations based on powders obtained from herbs such as spoonwort, nettles, and plantain, diluted in sweet liqueurs made from honey and "Syrian roses." Opiates were sold along with astringents for the gums, called "Stones for the Teeth," made of rock alum and ferrous sulfate. A "sympathetic stone" that "arrests toothache in an instant and prevents the teeth from rotting" met with great success. Vulnerary waters, or "traumatic waters," were general medicines sold for diseases of the mouth, supposedly effectual for every type of trauma and pain.

In order to attract wealthy buyers, some remedies sold for an extravagant price, encouraging the conviction that they contained precious and exotic ingredients. Toward the end of the eighteenth century, Chiara Masieri presented for examination to the Venetian College of Physicians a rare liqueur, derived from ancient alchemic recipes. The enterprising female quack declared that she had mixed "gold lime, philosophically dissolved," blended with the "finest Amber," and "Pearls, red and white Coral, ivory shavings and deer's horn," plus extracts of fine woods dissolved in "spirits obtained from roses and the liquid of honey."[6]

At the end of the eighteenth century, Angelo Faustini was awarded a license to sell his odontological specifics in Rome. A precursor of the modern theory of focal infection, he asserted that "the afflictions brought on by infirmities of the Teeth not only damage health, but can often cause Death." He declared that he could make false teeth that had "satisfied not only our domestic nobility, but foreign nobility as well." His prices were not exorbitant: Anyone who would "honor him at his shop, will pay only three pavoli; at [their] home, five pavoli; as for noblemen, he will be contented ... with their courtesy."[7]

The odontological prescriptions of illustrious physicians and academics, infused as they were with a vague flavor of sophistry, were not all that different from those of the quacks. Professor Vitali, a celebrated doctor whom we shall meet later, advised touching the aching tooth with the leg of a toad, or tying a small bit of plumbago, or leadwort, to the back of the hand before retiring in the evening: "[I]n the morning the hand is livid, and the pain gone."[8]

Tooth drawers did not disappear altogether from the scene until the beginning of the twentieth century; wandering practitioners carrying their instrument cases could still be found at country markets and fairs, right up to the time when dentistry became established as an honorable profession. In the second half of the nineteenth century, Renato Fucini described a charlatan named Bennati, who extracted teeth with a masterly stroke of his long, shining sword while sitting on his horse; his patients, mouths wide open, waited apprehensively in the midst of the crowd. During that same period a father and son named Trentuno became famous; these charlatans, armed with a large bag of pincers and tongs, pulled teeth on horseback, the suffering patient's head held firmly between their legs.

Three Special Characters

Three special characters enlivened Italian quackery in the eighteenth century: Though they were from different cultural and social backgrounds, they had many similar adventures and parallel experiences. Their exploits, recounted in lively autobiographies, illustrate the contradictory aspects of an era in transition, a time in which the Enlightenment's turmoil of ideas fostered the enterprises of the most able charlatans.

THE "ALFIER LOMBARDO"

Giuseppe Colombani wrote his remarkable memoirs in a small book, printed in 1724. Still an adolescent, he ran away from home and embarked as cabin boy on a merchant ship headed for Barcelona. He became adept at fencing, and his physical prowess, added to a talent for music and dancing made him popular with audiences everywhere.[9] His vocation for the life of a quack was revealed while he was in Sicily; he learned the first basics in Palermo, from an "Old Persian," a popular charlatan who, amazed at Colombani's expertise with swords, hired him to work with his company, even promising his daughter Angelica's hand in marriage in exchange for fencing lessons. Colombani's admiration knew no bounds after he had witnessed the old man drink a potent poison in front of his public. The Persian turned yellow and swelled up as though he were dying; then he swallowed his own powerful antidote before the stunned public, and by the next day he had miraculously returned to life and was able to sell more than two thousand jars of his wondrous antidote. These frauds, carefully invented, competently and adroitly executed, revealed the fascinating art of quackery to Colombani, who realized that the unerring success of a true charlatan lay in his capacity to convince his public.[10]

By this time, Colombani considered himself an expert in the art of fraud and decided that it was time for him to become independent. He abandoned Angelica and assumed the heroic name of "Alfier Lombardo" in memory of his native region. In Naples he became an immediate, clamorous success; at the theater, even the Viceroy applauded as he danced, sang, juggled, and interpreted the lead in an operetta for which he himself had composed the music. During the intervals, a colleague took charge of selling his prodigious medicinal remedies, and the money began to roll in.

His success was so phenomenal that he was able to earn "two thousand doubloons," which he swiftly squandered, traveling through France and England with Frine, a beautiful Spanish ballerina. His wandering came to an end when he returned to Italy; arriving in Leghorn, he met Apollonia, the daughter of an expert tooth drawer, who was to become his bride. With her urging, Colombani finally decided to abandon his deceits for good and began new experiences as a healer and tooth drawer, instructed by his wife, who was an expert dentist in her own right.

Apollonia convinced him to attempt the conquest of opulent Venice. They could not have chosen a better place to demonstrate their skills: The prosperous republic, a center for commerce and trade with vast terrestrial and maritime dominions, was a veritable paradise for charlatans. A swarm of people of every rank, a ceaseless, multihued, boisterous crowd of common folk and elegant patricians constantly passed through the square dedicated to Saint Mark, similar to an open-air parlor enclosed on three sides by columns with the shining mosaics of the great basilica serving as backdrop. Peddlers of "acque nanfe," distilled waters perfumed with orange blossom, glided through the throngs selling their wares. The flood of

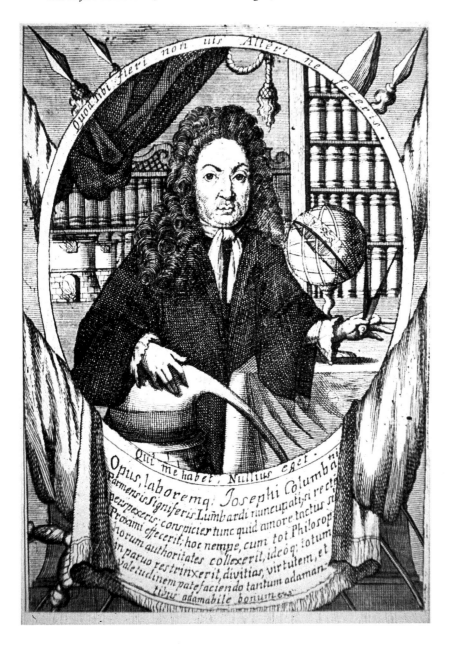

Portrait of the charlatan Giuseppe Colombani, alias the "Alfier Lombardo." The inscription in Latin at the bottom of the frame reads: *"Whoever has me, needs nothing else."* From Colombani's autobiography. Biblioteca Nazionale Centrale, Firenze.

humanity stopped in knots before players and singers, listened to storytellers illustrating the exciting, fantastic tales depicted on painted canvas,
halted before the puppet theaters to laugh at the jests of Punchinella and
Harlequin. In the midst of this lively confusion, small groups gathered to
hear the numerous charlatans who, with musical accompaniment, shouted
the properties of their remedies.

The Alfier set up his large stage, decorated with splendid banners and
surrounded by halberds; he played minuets with his trumpet and deftly
showed off his magnificent sword and his "pikes for war and tournament."
As soon as a large gathering had formed, the charlatan told of his expertise in "drawing, cleaning, implanting, and making false teeth," demonstrating his methods for "healing fluxions, curing ulcers, abscesses, and
fistulas."

The Alfier Lombardo practiced his trade for twenty-four years in the
elegant, teeming square, surrounded by the bustle of the "marketplace of
the world." He confessed that only his wife could outshine him in valor —
"a celebrity who sent to the Press in Venice, in 1719, a Labor in which she
takes the just defense of Women, demonstrating that they can be skilled
in Virtues, equal with men." Apollonia was a prodigious woman: On the
evening of November 25, 1723, before an astonished crowd, she pulled a
"monstrous" tooth after all the other tooth drawers had failed, demonstrating that women can be equal to men in surgical maneuvers that require
not only dexterity, but strength and self-control. She must have possessed
these gifts, for by her own confession, she had pulled more than five thousand teeth in her lifetime.[11]

Encouraged by his wife, the Alfier Lombardo became completely committed to his difficult profession and decided to abandon forever the fraudulent stratagems of his former errant life. The ambitious charlatan buried
himself in the study of medical books; learning and experimenting, he
discovered new remedies against pain and inflammation and became a
renowned expert in the art of tooth drawing. In a small volume, he illustrated the anatomy of the teeth and the maxillary bones without error,
along with "figures, and Instroments engraved in copper" that he had personally fashioned. The instruments that he used to bare the tooth and a
dental forceps of his own invention for extracting the roots were used as
dental surgical instruments until modern times. His transformation was
so profound, his regret so sincere that he wished to make amends by warning the public, urging his readers to keep their eyes open, for no one could
recognize his swindling colleagues better than he. Instead of repeating the
swagger and dishonesty of many of the tooth drawers in the squares, the
Alfiere warned his public that after an extraction many "ugly accidents"

could occur, especially if the tooth had deep roots that were "embraced and restricted, ... bound by many, many nerves."[12] He was now dedicated to fighting fraud in quackery, the art that had once fascinated him and that he knew well for having practiced it for so many years.

Although the claim that he had pulled half a million teeth during his lifetime is perhaps an exaggeration, the Alfier Lombardo was considered the most respected tooth drawer in the Venetian Republic; his success as a healer and expert, prudent surgeon was undeniable. He stated that sometimes, when he had cured a person from his suffering, the crowd, "crying hurrah, hurrah," carried him bodily home.

THE "UNKNOWN KNIGHT"

"The Marvelous Life of the Unknown Knight, Comedian, Swordsman, Hermit, Charlatan, and Surgeon dentist of the King of Sardinia," written around the end of the eighteenth century, is a ponderous autobiographical manuscript that recounts the adventures of Vittorio Cornelio.[13] The exploits of this charlatan faithfully mimic those of the Alfier Lombardo and once more tell of the progressive transformation of an equivocal character unhampered by scruples into a celebrated and highly regarded professional. Cornelio, like Colombani, was an expert swordsman and restless wanderer; his life was spent contriving swindles, getting into duels and brawls, and performing in theatrical exhibitions, but in the end his passion for anatomy and the art of medicine was so overwhelming that his worth became known and appreciated even in the academic circles of his city.

The story of the young Vittorio Cornelio is similar to that of other famous adventurers and charlatans of the period: He was born to a bourgeois family, but instead of studying, he preferred to travel and acquire new experiences. After a brief stint as an actor in a company of comedians, he applied himself to fencing and mastered the art so well that he became a teacher, even writing a small treatise on the subject.

He was suddenly smitten with irresistible fascination for a strange, histrionic sorcerer of unknown nationality and uncertain faith who surrounded himself with an aura of mysterious exoticism. Just as Colombani had been full of admiration for the old Persian, Cornelio was captivated by this other mysterious charlatan who called himself "Monsieur Pomer." "His fortunes were immense," Cornelio wrote with admiration: "The observations of plants, of minerals, and of the most notable antiquities were the purpose of his travels. Letters, credentials, licenses and privileges from the greatest sovereigns of Europe distinguished him everywhere.

From this famed teacher, Cornelio learned to prepare secret potions and, after a period of practicing the fundamental notions necessary to begin the practice of lithotomist on "sections of cadavers," to perform minor surgery.

Gifted with a clever tongue, he soon became such an artist that during an Easter pageant, "a warm and copious weeping wet the cheeks of the onlookers." In his autobiography he frankly recounts his amorous adventures with both sexes, including "Dear Maddalena," a lovely widow who died on the eve of their marriage; disconsolate, Cornelio abandoned the theater to drift from one religious shrine to another.

Cornelio made the decision to leave the career of actor for good; calling himself "Professor Dental Surgeon," he traveled all over the central and southern regions of Italy, performing innumerable feats of minor surgery with extraordinary success, but also often using every kind of swindle and fraud. At last, like every famous charlatan, he decided to make his entrance into Rome, and with the money that he had earned, he presented himself clothed in the most "noble and affluent magnificence." He writes that under his "fine black cape" he wore a vest on which hundreds of "double gold coins" shone. Because of this ostentatious pomp he ended up being robbed by an unfaithful servant, whom he fruitlessly chased as far as Civitavecchia. He spent the little money he had left to buy a charlatan's license and that same evening set up a platform in the main square, where he began, "by the light of two torches, to speak to the people." Instead of offering, as was the style of other charlatans, "some balsam from Arabia brought after my voyage to Jerusalem, or a specific carried from Spain," he exploited the pseudoscientific curiosity of the onlookers. After thunderous applause, he sold his concoctions with ample profit.[14]

Since it was the custom for charlatans to challenge each other with scientific arguments, the Unknown Knight's perfect knowledge of human anatomy came in very handy. He used this knowledge as a powerful weapon and won implacable arguments with his rivals in the public squares, convincing the last skeptics of his vast medical knowledge.

Traveling from one Italian city to another, one day the Unknown Knight reached Ancona; to his dismay, he discovered that he had been preceded by another celebrated charlatan, Giovanni Greggi, alias "The Cosmopolitan." This dangerous rival, who had arrived in town announced by the blaring of trumpets and the roll of kettledrums, had taken up residence in the best hotel in town, occupying "the most luxurious and grand apartments, ordinarily destined for the most respectable princes and eminent cardinals."

To demonstrate his magnificence and wealth, the Cosmopolitan invited the Unknown Knight to a sumptuous dinner, during which, "accompanied by the most exquisite liqueurs, choice dishes, and foreign wines," three concerts were performed — an unforgettable banquet that lasted more than three hours, served by "twenty-four servants grandly dressed in resplendent liveries." It was not lost on the Unknown Knight that his rival's splendid demonstration was a clever display, purposely designed to encourage him to abandon town. Not in the least deterred by his adversary, the next evening he appeared in the same square in which the Cosmopolitan was selling his "cephalic, antiputrid, disobstructing, balsamic, softening, febrifugal, and antivenereal balsam, valid for a hundred ills."

A memorable competition took place between the two charlatans: the Unknown Knight mounted his platform illuminated by "twelve torches, each with four wicks, and four silver candlesticks," but the Cosmopolitan "commanded his servants to make a deafening din with their instruments," in order to drown out his rival's voice and disrupt his entertainment. The Unknown Knight hoisted a movable skeleton and, with professional manner, resolutely began to illustrate his "anatomical reasonings." At this point his listeners, overcome with curiosity and interest, turned against the harassing musicians of the opposing company and smothered them with "loud whistling until they were obliged to hush."

"In possession of the field," recounts the Unknown Knight in his memoirs, "a universal silence fell, and I unloosened my tongue in the promise that each evening I would pledge myself to give lessons to the crowd." At that point, even his rival, surprised and curious, stopped to listen with all his retinue.

Once he was sure that the audience was completely in his hands after the amazing anatomical demonstrations, the Knight announced to the public that he was not the usual opportunistic, venal quack but a "veritable expert in human needs"; unlike his rival, who gloried in the possession of an arcane secret for all ills, he presented himself to the onlookers as a person profoundly erudite in the medical arts and interested in "investigating the nature of the disease before ordering the remedy."[15]

Finally abandoning cunning and trickery, Cornelio passed a difficult and lengthy examination with twenty interrogations, obtaining excellent marks and the sought-after license of surgeon-dentist. He began his practice in the square with his new title; in a short time, because of his experience and knowledge of the anatomy of the mouth, he gained enormous favor with the public.

At the bottom of his heart, the Knight was nostalgic for the life of a quack; how could he forget his glorious adventures, the long voyages, the risks overcome, the actor's disguises, the satisfaction, the amorous escapades, the money earned and lost, the daring operations and challenges in the open squares? "The work of a charlatan," he wrote, "is so open that it can be publicly judged as the ancient physicians did; and this is more honest and sincere than operating in private." Instead of pointing out all empirics for dishonor and infamy because of their chatter and impostures, he insisted that a distinction should be made between ability and ignorance, dependability and trickery, truth and deceit. He was convinced that "The most erudite and excellent professors of medicine spring from quackery." The empirical art "deserves credit and praise, for it is certain and sure, being based on experience," and its remedies are "the best, the most beneficial ... simple, of little cost, and enough to medicate an entire hospital."

In an imaginary debate with an anonymous critic who accuses charlatans, the Knight argues that this art is "not humbled for being mixed with singing, with clowns and other ridiculous personages and comic acts. If anything it is the eternal, continuous, bitter aversion of official medicine against charlatans that forces them to attract their audience with that which is pleasing or ridiculous."[16]

BONAFEDE VITALI: CELEBRATED DOCTOR AND MOUNTEBANK

The friendship between Carlo Goldoni and Bonafede Vitali was sealed over a steaming cup of chocolate. The famed playwright writes in his memoirs that he was in Milan in an especially depressed state of mind, having just burned his play "Amalasunta." He decided to pay a visit to Vitali, the well-known doctor-charlatan, mainly out of curiosity. "A personage of a very rare species," Goldoni amusedly wrote, "whose memory deserves to be recorded in the annals of the century." At their first encounter, the two conversed at length, and the playwright found in Vitali "much civility and graciousness of manner." He adds that "he was as pleasing in private as he was erudite in public."[17] Pretending that he wished to buy one of his famous remedies, Goldoni proceeded to reel off a list of his disturbances, mostly invented, but the amused professor soon saw through him and offered a cup of hot chocolate as the best cure for his ills.

Bonafede Vitali was unique in the history of medicine and charlatanism. He came from a very good family and had received an excellent education. The story of his restless life, including the usual bellicose interlude with a Venetian regiment, was written by a nephew after his death and is similar to that of other adventurous charlatans. After brilliantly obtaining a degree in medicine and chemistry, he participated in various clashes as army surgeon until he received a bayonet wound. On leaving the army, he traveled far and wide through Europe and as far as Russia; he later took up residence in England for several years, finding himself there during an epidemic of plague which raged throughout the country. Then, like Colombani, he took to sea, sojourning in the main ports of Spain and France. His career as charlatan began in Genoa, where he chose the name of "The Anonym," suggesting mystery and secrecy; he presented himself to the public, ready to "answer any question, and to discuss, and to dispute at length, any matter proposed." His profession wavered between a respectable medical practice and quackish exhibitions, and in both fields he obtained immense satisfaction.

"This singular man," Goldoni later wrote, "to whom no science was foreign, had an immoderate desire to make use of the whole of his knowledge; and since he was a better speaker than writer, he gave up the honorable position that he held, and took the resolution to become a mountebank and entertain the public; but, since he was not rich enough to be content with glory alone, he gained profit from his talent by selling his medicines. For him, the profession of quack was an excellent one; his specifics were good, and his science and eloquence earned him uncommon credit and esteem." The playwright remembers how he "publicly solved the most difficult matters in all the sciences and abstract matters that were brought to his attention. Problems, points of criticism, of history, of literature etc. were discussed on his empirical theater, and he held forth with the most satisfying dissertations."

Praise, honors, appointments offered by governments and universities were heaped upon him, as were requests for consultations: He gave advice to the physicians of the doges of Venice and Genoa, he was invited to the courts of King Charles XII of Sweden and Louis XIV of France. The grand duke of Florence, Gian Gastone de' Medici, grateful for some precious therapeutical advice, presented him with a splendid diamond; the Florentine College of Physicians hailed him as "master of science."

Vitali deemed experience to be the only true and legitimate medicine; he was a follower of an empirical art that refused secret theories, which were often used to hide ignorance of the cause of disease: This was a healthy empiricism, necessary to contrast the dominating theories of corrupt humors and the thoughtless misuse of bloodlettings, purges and enemas. Vitali felt that his professional respectability was in no way diminished by his preference for "exchanging the chair or the tribune for a quack's platform."[18] He practiced a simple medicine, born of practical observation learned from humble folk, the same as that of many famous charlatans who had preceded him, from Paracelsus to Fioravanti.

His good friend Scipione Maffei often urged him to give up his quack-ish activities, but Vitali answered him in an audacious pamphlet that challenges orthodox medicine, a declaration in favor of popular empiricism, in which Vitali explains that "the quack, if he behaves with honesty, is most useful to humanity, for his art is the result of salutary experience; in fact, only healthful empiricism will profitably remain in the history of medicine through the variations of all theories." He states with courage: "Many of those responsible for orthodox medicine will be judged as ignorant, and braggarts, and agents of fraud."[19] He recognizes that the spectacle, which amazes the crowds and provokes scorn in his be-robed colleagues, is indispensable for quacks, obliged to be accompanied by comic actors and buffoons for the sole purpose of claiming the public's attention. Instead of persecuting charlatans, it would be more appropriate to deny licenses to ignoramuses and others in whose "veins flow vile blood."[20]

Bonafede Vitali's renowned eloquence and the elegance of his speech were a necessary corollary for his performances in the squares and the practice of his art. Before the show, the actors busied themselves helping their employer collect the money, knotted in handkerchiefs, that the public threw on stage; the handkerchiefs were then thrown back, this time tied around little jars and boxes that contained various medicines. When the commercial phase was over, a play in three acts followed, "by the light of torches made of white wax, and with a certain similar magnificence." Naturally there was also a prima donna, who recited on the platform along with the Anonym.

A huge crowd of people on foot and in carriages filled the square wherever the doctor-quack performed, "and this new Hippocrat," Goldoni writes, "sold his remedies, and lavished his rhetoric, surrounded by the four masks of Italian comedy."[21]

Such was the friendly collaboration between playwright and doctor that two singers and a conductor, musicians in the merry, charlatanesque company of professor Vitali, performed a duet during the interlude in Goldoni's first successful comedy, "The Venetian Gondolier."

CHAPTER 10

A Carnival of Publicity

It may have been useless chatter that poured forth from the mouths of quacks, and yet, although loathed by physicians and apothecaries, threatened by magistrates, observed with suspicion by clerics and chased by bailiffs, their success was undeniable. "That army of brigands, possessing nothing, obtains all," wrote Pietro Aretino in a letter to the famous charlatan, Jacopo Coppa, in 1543. In his habitual bantering tone, Aretino professes his admiration for the clever Coppa: Convinced that no one is able to better persuade the public nor provide more publicity than a quick-witted charlatan, he begs him to use his "natural eloquence to ring out clearly before all" Aretino's name.[1]

Erudite but exasperated professors were perfectly aware of the success that ignorant quacks obtained with their cascades of words. In 1621, the jurist Paolo Zacchia threatened punishment for those who had the impudence to offer panaceas for ailments of all kinds by using "their certain natural and verbose eloquence."[2]

During the Counter-Reformation, the church often railed furiously against charlatans. The Jesuit priest Ottonelli wrote, "these wicked followers of the devil put on masks, climb onto platforms, tell lies, deceive simpletons and sell merchandise. No one believes them because they are liars, no one trusts them because they are false, and no person with a healthy mind and honest life stops to see their exhibitions." But even he was forced to admire their inexhaustible dialectic and admit that their renown depended more on their perspicacious and pleasing form of rhetoric than on the curative capacity of their remedies. Every vendor, he explained, needs the "histrionic artifice" of words, but this is not a gift possessed by all. Therefore a charlatan who is "not suited to enrapture Men with his voice" will not achieve success, and every attempt will fail miserably.[3] It was not sufficient to invent jokes or hire masks and players; a charlatan must know how to speak, how to convince his listeners; this was a gift of Nature that not all enjoyed. But with the availability of the printed word, charlatans were provided with a new and powerful means of advertising themselves, a means with which they could attract clients without being obliged to cry out in the public squares.

Bills of Invitation

Between the sixteenth and seventeenth centuries, the first notices or "bills of invitation," printed and distributed by quacks or their helpers, appeared: These were pages of various nature that were meant to be read out in public. For the benefit of those who were illiterate, and these were legion, there were hired assistants who read out loud, declaiming the excellence of the remedies and the merits of their employers.

Jacopo Coppa began his career as editor and distributor of handbills. The celebrated charlatan, who must have possessed some learning, would read out loud at the top of his voice the most significant passages, combining the sale of these booklets with the vending of cosmetics, soaps, and miraculous specifics.

Toward the end of the eighteenth century, a Florentine cleric found a frayed booklet containing several loose sheets on which the expenses of the printing shop of the ancient monastery of Saint Jacob in Ripoli had been noted in the fifteenth century. Many orders came from charlatans, who bought prayers, pieces of the New Testament, Sunday aphorisms, and simple popular poems. Many charlatans paid with lira or a few florins at the time of ordering; others left "a tablecloth" as pledge or promised to settle their account with "half a stack of oak logs."[4]

Bills were posted on corners, on columns, or in the city markets; the authorities rarely intervened, even when physicians and apothecaries protested against the advertisements. "Flagellum demoniorum," "very powerful against Demons and Spells of any kind, against temptations, fevers, headache, pain in childbirth, worms," and an indispensable protection against "dangerous encounters," was one exception: It was banned, and the bills were torn from the walls because of the firm opposition of the religious authorities, who judged that it encouraged a dangerous form of superstition.

"The great virtues, and marvelous effects of the Liqueur" called "Philosophical Oil" could be examined in the handbill of an anonymous charlatan: a liqueur that "benefits frigid, humid, and windy stomachs" insuperable as a cure for "anxiety, vapors of the head, and trembling of the heart, apoplexy, hemorrhoids or piles, birthing pains, quartan fevers." The charlatan warns not to place it near "lighted lamps, for it is liquor, that attracts flame to itself as a magnate does iron, and will burn, and could cause great damage"; a timely warning, for to calm stomach pains, the patient was instructed to spread it on his "staff."[5]

Some doctors had no qualms about imitating the hated quacks' methods of sales promotion. One of them, who presented himself as Doctor Balanzon, was a scion of the Castiglione family, esteemed physicians who operated in the area of Milan during the seventeenth century. He distributed a handbill which advertised many "natural and academic secrets," along with advice on every subject, from beauty aids, to powders that would eliminate rats and lice, and even instructions for organizing social entertainments and "conversational games."[6]

Gazettes

Gazettes provided charlatans with an unexpected means of advertising and exonerated them from having to entertain the public with talk. This new and original form of propaganda appealed to a public that belonged to a more elevated, though not less credulous, social rank.

In the beginning, the gazettes were not widely regarded, and life was not easy for many newspaper hacks; some of them, found to be too curious and interested in other peoples' business, were persecuted and imprisoned. In the kingdom of Naples a few were even hanged, accused of having divulged "facts shaming some Gentlemen" or having written "obscene and heretical things."

Italy was the first European state to print important news in the gazettes, intended for merchants about to embark on their travels: economical opportunities offered by different states, perils that could derive from war or the continuous shifting of political situations. Mail masters, couriers, story writers, informers, deliverers and newsboys were charged with distributing these newspaper sheets, which took their name from the "gazzetta," a Venetian coin worth three soldi.

By the middle of the eighteenth century, the *Gazzetta Toscana*, official organ of the grand duchy, had acquired a substantial circulation and a good number of readers. It printed official notifications, news of the arrival of ambassadors and major prelates, announcements of holidays, celebrations and ceremonies and the births, weddings and deaths of illustrious personages, besides informing of the arrivals of ships and the movements of goods. The gazettes often printed occasional news of a clearly servile cast: Sometimes it informed that a sovereign or the Holy Father had received benefit from bloodletting; occasionally it even went as far as to indicate their favorite purge, "if mustard or rather rhubarb to keep in good health."[7]

The *Gazzetta Toscana* in 1773 published an announcement by "Doctor" Giovanni Vannini, who lists his address in Florence as "across the street from the Marquis Bartolomei." With professional seriousness, he claims to possess a secret that will cure all kinds of cancer. If the cure should fail by rare chance, as consolation and for the "delight of the patient," he promises to "demonstrate a Machine of transparent Crystal, representing Saint Peter in Rome, which is one of the most beautiful things ever seen of this type." Success must not have been lacking, for he repeated the same advertisement in the Tuscan newspaper for several months at his own expense.[8]

A pompous declaration by Giovanni Cleri, "apothecary of the Noble College of Rome," was published for "Lovers of Medical Innovations" in a small insert sold with the newspaper; it has all the appearance of a sly ploy invented by two dishonest pharmacists. Cleri confesses to the readers, in a fawning introduction, that not even the "strictest laws of friendship" can force him to conserve the secret of a specific discovered by his colleague, a "princely apothecary" from Modena; this specific is an infallible cure for epilepsy, a horrendous disease that even physicians call "obrobrium medicorum." He describes a young man, smitten with the tragic malady, who fell prey to terrible convulsions, uttering screams so "frightening as to inspire terror into the onlookers," and causing his poor parents to be disconsolate. After the first dose of specific, the convulsions ceased, and after a month's cure he returned to his former robust and healthy constitution. The incredible recovery was confirmed under oath and certified by a notary in front of various witnesses.[9]

The medical profession tried to react against this scandalous type of advertising, but with limited success, for they had only the newly born medical publications at their disposition. On the introductory page of "Il Giornale di Medicina," the first Italian medical journal, printed in Venice in 1763, the publisher unleashed a tirade against charlatans, their secret cures, and the public's gullibility.

The *Gazzetta Toscana* offered charlatans an invaluable chance to attract the public's attention; most advertisements were paid for, but a few were free of charge; these last exalted the works of particular healers and were composed by the editorial staff, usually upon pressure by an authority or after the personal approval of the grand duke. The privilege was reserved for charlatans of indisputable skill: tooth drawers, lithotomists, and oculists of undeniable fame. Often the articles that announced the arrival in town of a charlatan were printed in bolder type that those that reported a fortunate cure performed by a physician or the successful operation of some surgeon.

Italy was the preferred destination of the most celebrated English charlatan of the eighteenth century, "Chevalier" John Taylor, oculist to King George II. Taylor was an able eye surgeon who managed to combine quackery with unequaled courage and impudence. He knew the anatomy of the eye better than most and possessed an indisputable manual ability, using instruments that he had invented himself.

For his detractors, and they were legion, his success was due to the peremptory orders given to his patients: They were bid to keep their eyes bandaged for several days after the operation; before any errors could become apparent, Taylor had vanished. It seems that hundreds of patients became definitively blind after he operated on them, although the times and the conditions in which he worked must be held in mind. Nonetheless, Taylor became one of the most renowned eye surgeons of his century and at the same time one of the most debated, pointed out either in admiration or contempt. Horace Walpole refused a letter of recommendation to Taylor for a friend about to depart for Rome: "We are not conscious of any such merit, nor have any of our eyes ever wanted to be put out."

Even if his fame and his skill unleashed the envy and scorn of most of the English medical establishment, he obtained considerable success with foreign doctors and was held in high esteem by French and German oculists. As his name became established all over Europe, many foreign universities conferred doctoral titles upon him. The fortunate and daring quack perfected the technique of extracting cataracts, a technique that had not made much progress since the time of the Egyptians. He succeeded in smashing the crystalline lens with special instruments, pushing it into the vitreous humor of the eyeball. It is not certain that he ever attempted the modern technique of extraction with success, although he mentions it in one of his writings.

Nichols, in "Literary Anecdotes of the Eighteenth Century," describes how Taylor performed one of his celebrated operations: "The doctor appeared dressed in black with a light, flowing, ty'd wig; ascended a scaffold behind a large table raised about three feet from the ground and covered with an old piece of tapestry on which was laid a dark coloured cafoy chariot seat with four black bunches (used upon hearses) tyed to the corners for tassels, four large candles on each side of the cushions and a quart decanter of drinking water with a half pint glass to moisten his

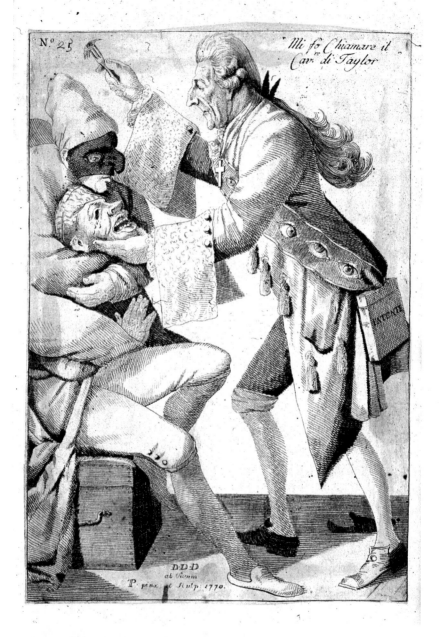

Caricature of the famous English charlatan John Taylor, his coat decorated with eyes, holding a patient's eye triumphantly on a fork. Thomas Patch (1710). Biblioteca Nazionale Centrale, Firenze.

mouth." Some of his other operatory exhibitions concerned squint and daring plastic surgery. Without anesthesia, he cut the subcutaneous skin of a woman's eyelid, which had been so disfigured by a burn that she was unable to close it. When the woman screamed in pain, he cried out, "Remember Lady: Beauty! Beauty!" giving her the courage to continue the operation, which apparently had a fortunate outcome.[10]

An article, so far gone unnoticed by Taylor's biographers, appeared in the first issues of the "Gazzetta Toscana" of 1769, informing readers of the imminent arrival in Florence of the oculist chevalier Giovanni De Taylor; the "De" had been added in Italy to give his name an aura of nobility. The journal announces his arrival as it would that of a celebrity, stressing that he comes "from Bologna, where he performed many difficult operations…; abiding only a few days, for he must go, because invited, to Rome, having been called by a gentleman of lofty condition."

Once the famous oculist had settled himself at the "Black Eagle," one of the best inns in Florence, the gazette again announced that "the Cavalier Giovanni De Taylor, Oculist, Papal, Royal and Electoral, well known in all of Europe for the number of his operations no less than for his mastery and skill in the art of curing diseases of the eye, will remain for a few days, devoting himself to helping those many people who have come here from different countries." The reporter invites the entire population, but especially the nobility, to be present at De Taylor's operations and observe his surgical instruments.[11]

Taylor was proficient in several languages; he called his oratory "true Ciceronian, a prodigiously difficult style never before attempted in our language." He was handsome and known to be a womanizer and incorrigible suitor; like Casanova, he was not shy about recounting his amorous adventures in many European countries. He was particularly attracted by young nuns, whom he called his "religious beauties." He even wrote a small volume in Italian, on "How to Make Love with Success." No copies of the book exist; they were probably burned by the Italian editor, who may have been nervous about its offensive content, but its loss to posterity most probably does not represent an irreparable deprivation for literature.

Medical and Cosmetic Remedies

In their advertisements, many charlatans combined the sale of medicines with that of prodigious cosmetic secrets. In the Florentine capital, "Baron" De' Girelli offered "soapy water" for the beard, a "sympathetic ball" for sharpening razors, and "sultanate water" to make the skin soft, but his most astounding secret, "born from his great perspirations and vigils," was contained in a mixture that would "make hair grow on those who are bald, and make hair fall out on those who have too much." However, the baron had to contend with a rival, a "professor chemist," who declared that, after lengthy studies, he had discovered two secrets that were even more ingenious: "one to make hairs fall out," the other which would "make hair grow and spring up as desired: black, brown, or blond."[12]

Medical quacks were not the only ones who advertised health remedies. "A cloth printer," who had his shop in Piazza dei Cimatori, offered his modest secret for only "ten coins an ounce"; this particular remedy was "a paste cooked in the oven, which, if tasted in small quantity by the Rat, instantly dies, and if tasted by any other Animal comes to no harm, on the contrary, eaten by men it becomes a cordial medicine."[13]

An announcement of aristocratic bent tells of the treatment undergone by Signor Francesco Pieraccini's daughter, who suffered from scrofula, "miraculously cured by the Count of Albany, by the special grace conserved in his illustrious family."[14]

Not infrequently, doctors themselves sold balsams and pills with portentous healing virtues. An esteemed medical officer of the Tuscan Regiment was not content with his miserable stipend: having made up his mind to retire, he commenced the sale of his "holy balsam," the same name as the one sold by "the Anonym," a fellow townsman whose good fortune he hoped to emulate.[15]

Not only powders, but certain pills became the fashion all over Europe: "pilule melagogae" to drain the bile and "hystericae opiatae" to calm the nerves. A Florentine doctor, Martelli, sold pills which he unimaginatively called "pillole Martelliane"; they were reputed to be excellent against venereal disease, or any tertian fever. Those who must "resort to writing" are requested to specify if the tertian fever is simple or double; in the latter case, the price will also be double.[16]

The enterprising widow of Auguste Belloste, celebrated physician and first surgeon of Madame Royal of Savoy, lost no time after her husband's death: In a letter to the public, she declared that she possessed the secret of Doctor Belloste's famous pills, with which he had obtained many incredible healings, including that of a libertine abbot who had developed syphilis. It was a secret that anyone could have easily arrived at, for the main component of the remedy was only mercuric salt.[17]

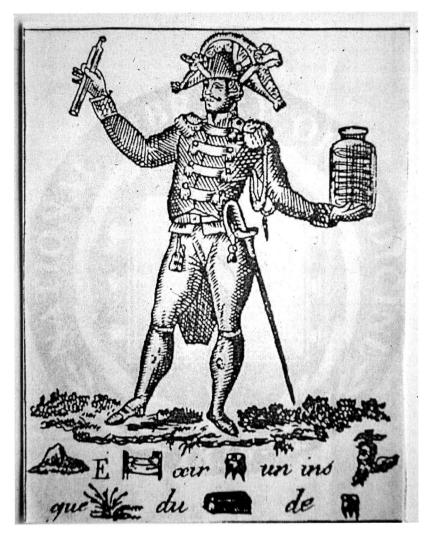

A French charlatan advertising his elixir against toothache. A rebus certifies "Mon elixir dans un instant guérit du mal de dents." U.S. National Library of Medicine, Bethesda, MD.

A Priest's Remedy for Ringworm

Charlatans had a particularly difficult time overcoming competition from monks and friars, for men of the church easily obtained the support of eminent and powerful figures to help the sale of their remedies.

"Tigna capitis," or ringworm, is an infection caused by a fungus that attacks the scalp; the disease was considered a grave misfortune, distressing and embarrassing for adults and children. Cures were useless, painful or dangerous, and transmission of the disease, because of a general promiscuity, was frequent. The only option was endurance: "La tegna che i la ga se la tenga" ("Whoever gets ringworm, keeps it") was a saying amongst the Venetian populace; Sicilians, considering that the available medical cures were worse than the disease, philosophically advised the afflicted person to keep his cap on his head, to avoid being discovered and laughed at. Hair removal was the only, even if temporary, remedy; one brutal system was to cut the sufferer's hair to about an inch in length, then put a leather cap, in which tar or resin had been spread, on his head. Once the sticky substance had taken hold, the victim was made to stand on a stool, the cap was tied to the ceiling, and, as in a hanging, the stool was kicked out from under him. The patient ended up on the ground, and the cap remained hanging from the ceiling with all the hair attached to it.[18]

A peculiar official notice appeared on the first page of the *Gazzetta Toscana* in the year 1774: The grand duke, Pietro Leopoldo, offered his lofty patronage to a cure for ringworm discovered by the Reverend Benedetto Forzoni Accolti, parish priest of Saint Clement in the town of Pelago. The reverend in turn declared that he had received it through the confidence of a "very erudite naturalist arriving from India." When the grand duke in person, along with his archiater and other distinguished doctors, was able to observe its "beneficial effects in divers subjects with Ringworm, the royal compassionate Heart was moved to acquire this medicament, unknown in Italy." After "generously remunerating the aforesaid Parish Priest," His Highness decided that "the said specific be rendered public, as well as the manner of use."

The gazette published the cunning priest's recipe in its entirety. As far as swindles go, it was in no way inferior to any charlatan's: "Take live frogs, put them in a glazed pot, and cover tightly.... Put the pot in a hot oven several times until the said frogs are well dried and cold." Once the frogs have been reduced to powder in a mortar, "grease the patient's head with pig's lard, and powder the head with the said powder, put over this a compressed pig's Bladder, cover the head with a cloth, and bandages so that the powder stays and remains applied to the head, and keep the medicament for 24 hours, then remove the bandages, take off the said bladder, and the patient will remain clean without any damage or pain." The lubrications were to be repeated for several days, until the "bulbs of the uprooted Ringworm" were eliminated.[19]

Frog's flesh was an ingredient that was not only used by quacks, but by official pharmacopoeia; according to a diffused belief, the blood of this animal healed, or at least halted, the progression of tubercular scrofula; it was sufficient to wear a string soaked in its blood.

From ancient times, an adverse fate seemed to mark every therapy for "tigna capitis": at the beginning of this century, the cures could be even worse. When it was discovered that radioactive substances had an energetic depilatory effect, a "modern" treatment was devised that involved putting a helmet of radium needles over the patient's head. The loss of hair was usually followed by local damage, necrosis of the scalp and often irreversible lesions to the hemopoietic system, especially in young patients. A photograph from the Alinari archives documents the brand-new therapy offered by radiation technology: A small patient affected with ringworm, assisted by an elegant nurse, is placed without any protection under a large radiferous helmet while a severe and bearded professor stands nearby, gravely supervising the dangerous treatment.

CHAPTER 11

"Physical Recreations"

The Golden Age of Quackery

The Age of Enlightenment soon became the Age of Gold for charlatans, a period of good fortune for many clever merchants of remedies. No other time in European history had seen such an invasion of quacks, nor had a similar degree of arrogance and pushiness been displayed by hordes of peddlers, secretists, medicasters, alchemists, adventurers and pseudoscientists who all used the sale of medicines as a springboard for their frauds.

Those who practiced the art of quackery had learned that it is impossible to fool a man without first pleasing him; any form of amusement or entertainment was helpful to attract the public. A magniloquent speech was usually preceded by comic actors in costume, music, singing, or farcical monologues; after the intermission, the actor, the buffoon, the mask abruptly changed countenance and became an expert in healing who could propose every kind of remedy.

In an age in which form was considerably more important than substance, charlatans were careful not to neglect their attire; the more extravagant appeared in three-cornered hats adorned with fluttering feathers, their breasts decorated with gold medals. Vasari had noted a century earlier: " Brocade coats, capes all embellished with gold cloth, the richest caps, necklaces, and similar other bagatelles, all things worthy of buffoons and mountebanks."[1] Many wore robes of red cloth with wide sleeves like the attire of learned doctors, which caused the Colleges of Physicians to protest; the provost of Bologna, at the end of the seventeenth century, began judicial proceedings against impudent rogues who "ofttimes mount platforms with dishonor and ridicule of true Physicians in doctoral robes."[2]

In Tuscany and the northern states, many charlatans wore a long black tunic in the manner of men of law, bedecked with lace and bright-colored braid and decorated in the most ostentatious manner possible. "But," thundered Professor Tissot, "despite their splendid appearance, with which many appear in public, they are nonetheless vile people."[3]

A long list of diplomas and testimonials of gratitude, either bona fide or false, granted by the most famous courts of Europe, and privileges conferred by nobles, popes, and royalty were exhibited on the lavishly furbished stage. While criers, with stentorian voices, praised the unbounded thaumaturgical merits of the charlatan and enumerated the awards that he had received from every part of the globe, pages distributed handbills on which the charlatan advertised his wares.

Large open-air medical fairs were certainly nothing new: For centuries the sale of solutives (purges), plasters, unguents, balsams, pills, oils, elixirs, stomachals, juleps, herbal mixtures, antidotes for poison, electuaries fortified with false gems, and precious hyacinths were a form of merry popular entertainment at fairs, in the squares and markets, at crossroads, in churchyards, in small villages, often even at the courts of the noblest palaces.

Compared to the sententious pronouncements of solemn physicians who insistently ordered torrential enemas, drastic emetics, exhausting purges and pitiless bloodlettings, the charlatans, from their small outdoor shops, offered pleasant remedies of herbal origin, almost always innocuous, accessible to all pockets. Was it not preferable to be consoled by these mysterious potions, to trust in these inoffensive and inexpensive cures, rather than resort to the great, haughty, presumptuous physicians of the century?

The public, inquisitive and amused, often with veiled complicity, delighted in the charlatans' witty quips and fanciful pantomimes, the sly winks and ironical barbs directed at the vain and peremptory pronouncements of learned doctors. Orthodox medicine, torn between opposing and abstruse theories, was not only impotent to cure and put everyone in a bad humor, but it was out of tune with the public's frivolous curiosity. In spite of Professor Tissot's baleful predictions and terrifying writings, people seemed to prefer the playful, satisfying and hopeful cures proposed by quacks, who promised not only health, but renewed youth and lasting beauty.

The charlatan's generosity seemed to have no limit: not only did he offer cheaply those remedies which ordinarily only the wealthy could afford, but displaying magnificence and munificence, he often proffered his precious, secret arcane free to the public — perhaps not all, but at least a "small quantity contained in a box." Almost always there was a solemn promise that the money spent to buy the remedy would be entirely refunded if the cure did not succeed: a good-natured deception that the crowd, after witnessing an elegant and entertaining spectacle without paying, willingly accepted. Even Scipione Mercuri, one of the most tenacious enemies of charlatans, had to recognize despite himself that charlatans' remedies were purchased even by those "who know they have been duped, as long as they make him keep acting the clown."[4]

The charlatan knew that the suggestion caused by his enchanting speech would soon vanish, but when the incautious victim awoke, he would be far away. His uninterrupted wandering ensured him easy impunity, infallibly ensured by the fact that no one likes to admit having been duped. The charlatan realized full well that he lived in a world of constant challenge and deceit, where fraud was not necessarily always on his part. If, with clever stratagems, he achieved some success, he would not only become rich, but would gain intimate satisfaction. Some went beyond every limit: An impudent charlatan, introducing himself as a "German doctor," claimed that he possessed the universal talisman, the definitive arcane, "indispensable for curing even those diseases for which physicians have not yet found a name."

These likable adventurers were favored by the public's irrepressible desire to possess any novelty, any remedy that was endowed with magical and extraordinary powers, even if the explanation was vague and impenetrable to reason. The charlatans' promises were only an extension of what people really desired for their own well-being, something that reality and intellect had always denied: It was an attempt by the medicine of the poor and the ignorant to affirm itself against that of the rich and powerful. The people's deeply rooted certainty that the medicines offered by erudite physicians were useless, drove deluded and abandoned patients to search desperately for any available help; the unscrupulous charlatans took advantage of the emotions and gullibility of the public, surrounding themselves with an aura of innovation, pseudoscience and mystery. Many pretended to be eccentric and extravagant travelers newly arrived from faraway countries, possessors of secret panaceas that would cure "a hundred and another thousand ills." The common opinion was that anyone who had traveled long and far must surely possess great experience and might even have discovered wonderful secrets and universal remedies.

In the mid-seventeenth century, a Sienese painter, Bernardino Mei, depicted a popular charlatan at work in the Piazza del Campo in Siena: an impressive man, hefty, bearded, seated on a large armchair. He wears an ample tunic tied at the waist in the oriental fashion with a sash of multi-

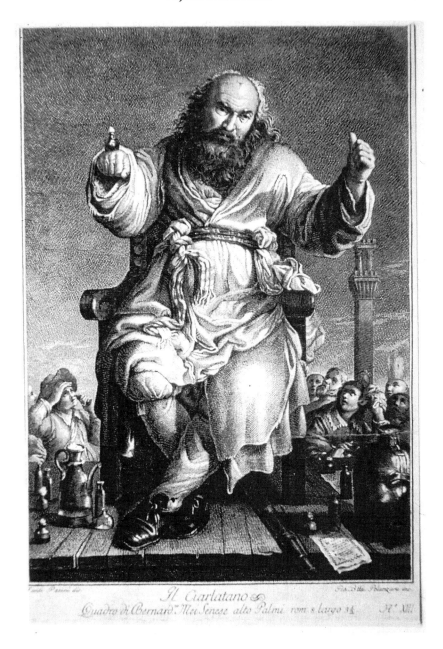

A charlatan in Siena. The quack holds up a small bottle with his miraculous cure. A telescope at his feet indicates that he is a man of science. Print by G.B. Polanzani and S. Pacini from the painting *The Charlatan* by Bernardino Mei (1636). Courtesy of Count Andrea Pannocchieschi D'Elci, Siena.

colored cloth. The charlatan has a piercing stare and a star-shaped scar on his forehead, which gives him an almost hieratic look; only his worn shoes betray his lowly condition and constant need to wander. From the height of his platform, this strange and disquieting person seems to dominate the crowd of common folk that press around him: They are painted looking up in fascination, mouths agape, inquisitive and shy, as he balances on the back of his hand a small, colored phial containing a precious medicinal liqueur. At his feet, beside a jumble of small bottles and phials of every shape and size, lies a rudimentary telescope; the very possession of this brand-new, mysterious instrument of science is motive for curiosity and attraction.

With the passage of time, many healers and nostrum mongers began to realize that their bizarre disguises, entertaining masques, parades of clowns and recitals with comic actors were by now suited only for the less shrewd inhabitants of the countryside and small towns; tricks with poisons and exhibitions with snakes had to give way to the more recent educational entertainments that the charlatans were quick to create, exploiting the amazing techniques of the newborn sciences.

The Enlightenment soon became a period of pseudoscientific quackery. The discovery of new and exciting phenomena produced by electricity, magnetism and other physical sciences such as chemistry and optics were transformed, in the minds of the public, into marvels that replaced ancient magic based on astrology and alchemy. By now the ignorant and often, even in the wealthier ranks of society, illiterate public was dominated by curiosity and the obsessive desire to try out the newest discoveries of the physical sciences. It must not be forgotten that more than half the male and three-quarters of the female population could not read or write; most of the others could barely do so. In the midst of this fervor, this insatiable desire for the modern and the marvelous, pretense and insolent fraud filled the spaces left empty by many unsolved scientific enigmas; a perfect opportunity for charlatans and quacks who, always in step with society's transformations, were ready to satisfy peoples' desires and dreams.

To further the sale of their specifics, charlatans now presented themselves as popular scientists, following up their speeches with powerful and stupefying experiments based on magnetism or electricity, or sometimes chemical amusements. Many of these "physical recreations" were part of charlatanesque prestidigitation: Pyrotechnical experiments in chemistry, games with phosphorus, enchantments constructed with air, water, electricity and magnetism were used to generate wonder and marvel. The prodigies of optics became a powerful means of visual persuasion; many quacks amused their audiences with shadow pictures, magic lanterns, boxes with a hole through which the eye could delight in a spectacle of animated drawings representing people and animals. Charlatans became artists and artisans of falsehood, modest manipulators of illusion, experts at presenting attractions that captured the audience's imagination, making it easier for them to cast their bait. The critical voices that branded these fabricators of deception as persons without shame whose final aim was to sell their remedies met with little success. In his *Cyclopedia*, in 1728, Chambers points out with disdain the ignorant quacks "who practiced low-level medicine without proper education or comprehension of the most fundamental principles of the art," and who with their false scientific reality took advantage of the lack of any critical sense on the part of the crowds. "They are nothing but clumsy imitators of Zoroaster," the acclaimed father of magic, who used science to teach "magnificent and astounding effects."[5]

Telescopic "Cannons" and "Minuscule Worms Full of Spirit"

People were fascinated by enlarged images that offered amazing visions hitherto unknown; if Galileo's telescopic "cannon" had permitted him to study the movements of the stars and the planets, the same instrument used "backward" became a means of bizarre entertainment. Thus, from the celestial marvels of the immensely distant, it was possible to enter into the wondrous phantasmagoria of the invisible.

The microscope, this "prodigious amplifier," as Jean Antoine Nollet, "electrician" of Louis XV enthusiastically declared, is "capable of transforming flies into sheep"; before the very eyes of bemused guests at court spectacles, he showed enormous flies and huge bees; tiny worms, invisible to the naked eye, squirmed incessantly beneath the lens. By now it was the conviction that many secrets of human existence could be unveiled by this instrument, a technical bewitchment that brought messages from another world. Metaphorically, enlargement became a sign of broadmindedness, as an irrational and limited outlook was associated with myopia.

Charlatans, attracted by the success in Germany and France of several booklets that explained the recondite preparation of "microscopic amusements," immediately grasped that the instrument could provide a way to draw crowds. By now, all over Europe, countless quacks used instruments copied from the real ones that were employed in experiments of physical science. The public's mania for instruments prompted an unidentified jester to make a counterfeit "microscopic falsometer," also called an "anaphorascopic flatterometer": a contraption complicated to an extreme, a towering structure covered with mirrors, lenses, tubes, prisms, glasses and regulating screws. It served for absolutely nothing except to make fun of those who admired every sort of complex contraption.

In 1740, M. Astruc, professor of medicine at the Royal College of France and consulting physician to the King, with the intention of unmasking charlatans, tells an amusing episode that had taken place in Paris in 1726. It was the dawning of the age of the microscope: Redi and Vallisnieri had already noticed "minuscule worms but full of spirit," in rotten meat, ciliates derived from putrefaction, tiny creatures that by "biting and gnawing" were assumed to be the cause of many of the diseases that distressed humanity. A charlatan by the name of Boile announced to a vast public his discovery that all diseases are caused by the little animals present in human blood; every type of disease is caused by a particular species of these pernicious little beings; fortunately, other minuscule animals could be unleashed to destroy them, "like hunting dogs destroy hares, or like vultures kill pigeons"—a method of cure that was "very sure, very brief, and very efficacious."

Boile declared that he had found out where the little rescuing creatures hid. To demonstrate the correctness of his theory, he used a special microscope that he had made himself. Instead of only one tube, it had five. To illuminate them all, he used various angled mirrors, which made the complicated instrument look more like a telescope than a microscope. At the distal extremity of one tube he placed a slightly concave glass that contained a few drops of blood serum taken from a patient. When the eyepiece was focused, an infinity of little beings, swimming around at high speed, appeared to the eye of the beholder. Once the dumbfounded public had been shown these innocuous little beasts, the charlatan put a few drops of another liquid, said to contain the helpers that would kill the enemy, on the concave glass. When the eyepieces were adjusted, the scene changed abruptly: the baneful little animals were all gone, annihilated by the good ones.

"Many people were dupes of these conjuring tricks," Astruc recorded. On critical examination it appeared evident that four of the microscope's five tubes did not serve for observation, but were essential for the ingenious fraud. Only one eyepiece was necessary, and the charlatan, by moving the container of tiny innocuous animals, could make the creatures that swam in the liquid appear or disappear at will. Astruc is indignant: "I know not what the charlatan hoped from his tricks," the good doctor wrote, "but I have learned that he had the prudence to avoid with flight the punishment that he deserved; having determined that his imposture was about to be discovered, he packed his bags and disappeared.... The hollow souls who had believed him admitted that they had been deceived, and thus in the end Medicine was happily vindicated."[6]

Perhaps an opportunity was lost, for no one ever thought, as a scientific hypothesis, to investigate the ingenious charlatan's expedient; involuntarily, he had preceded with his fantasies the discovery of microbes by a century and had predicted, with his fertile imagination, the destruction of pathogenic germs by white blood cells. Nonetheless, Boile's "discovery" deserved a tribute, and a reconstruction of his celebrated microscope remains as his memorial in the museum of the History of Medicine in Rome.

"Electrical Remedies"

Along with optics and chemistry, electricity offered the possibility of exciting and marvelous diversions. Ludovico Antonio Muratori, well-known man of letters, remembered an interesting encounter in 1746 with a wandering charlatan who demonstrated the thrill of electric "shocks." Muratori witnessed the show as he was passing one day in a square and was so enchanted that he commented, "[E]lectricity has revealed to us a new world and unveiled a secret exceedingly marvelous," adding, "That miraculous shaking" could offer medicine a "permanent healing of certain infirmities." "In my life I have never seen a thing surprise me more," Muratori wrote. "[F]rom an iron chain held by several arms one feels as a needle puncturing one's arm ... little flames jump out and the electrified man, who holds a naked sword in his hand, makes a flame appear at its point."[7] This particular quack was also mentioned in the Florentine "Literary Tales" as a "practical experimenter and wandering philosopher." Shocks were by now a miracle, a fascinating and mysterious enticement for the public.

In the eighteenth century, electricity was already used as a cure for various ailments. In 1779 Jean Paul Marat, a doctor who became notorious for unfortunate reasons, maintained that the human body was "subjected both to the action of atmospheric electricity and to that of organic, or innate, electricity resulting from the rubbing of the bones and nerves against the fluids and the muscles." For this reason he advised curing feverish patients with positive electricity during febrile shivers but with negative electricity in cases of hyperthermia.

In London, at the end of the last century, "Count" Mattei, a charlatan of Neapolitan origin, presented his prestigious "electrical remedies."

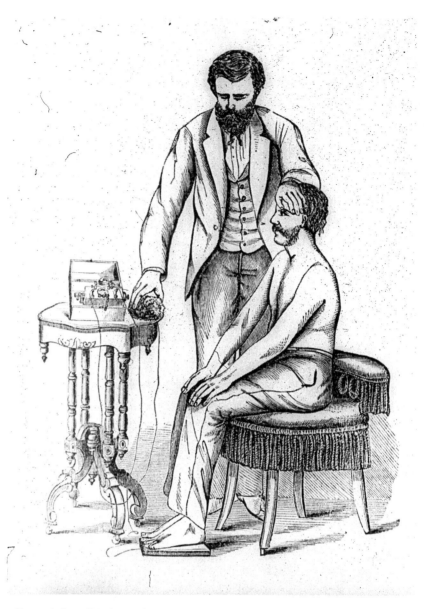

Xilograph from "A Practical Treatise on Medical and Surgical Uses of Electricity."
G. Beard, New York, 1881. U.S. National Library of Medicine, Bethesda, MD.

This "foreign nobleman" vowed that he could cure cataracts, broken bones, or any other ailment that malign nature had managed to conceive, with electricity. Within a short while he had plastered every location in the city with publicity: Advertisements announcing his remedy, bottled in three small colored phials full of "White, Red, and Green Electricity," in memory and gracious homage to the flag of his native land, appeared in newspapers, were posted on walls, in the streets, on omnibuses and trains, in the stations and even in public baths. At first, his success was clamorous, but it was abruptly interrupted by a curious doctor who analyzed the contents of the phials: It was discovered that the solution did not contain any electrical or magnetic properties at all, but only water. Shortly afterward, a London newspaper offered a useful suggestion to anyone wanting to become rich in a hurry: Buy a thousand gallons of water from the Thames for one pound and resell it, like Count Mattei, at five pounds an ounce.[8]

"Combustible" Man

The trick is described in the charlatan Falloppio's book: "To make a man look on fire, without swooning." The recipe is not very complicated: "[T]ake marshmallow and mix with whites of egg and spread with this any limb you wish: let it dry and then take sulfur powder ... and throw it in the fire, and it will burn without damage to the limb.... [Y]ou can touch the fire and you will not feel it." Even Garzoni, who is usually skeptical, mentions Lo Scoto Piacentino, who was able to "make a fire be born with marvelous effects."[9] Garzoni is forced to admit that sometimes "many professors of secrets" can reproduce extraordinary occurrences, leading common folk to believe that they are creators of miracles, but for the most part these are "mere illusions, and manifest deceptions, like those of charlatans."

Around the middle of the eighteenth century, a sensational event occurred which led scientists to reach improbable conclusions and several celebrated authors to invent morbid stories. A sixty-year-old noblewoman, Countess Cornelia Zagari nei Bardi from Cesena, heretofore in excellent health, was found one morning by her maid, four paces from her bed: Nothing was left of her but her legs and half of her arms; her trunk and most of her head had been reduced to smoking ashes. Unaccountably, neither the candles beside her bed, nor the sheets, nor the curtains had been burned. Beside her remains was an oily, sticky liquid whose nauseating odor had penetrated the rooms nearby. Several doctors and scientists decided that the cause was supernatural, others blamed a sulfur mine beneath her house, still others a stroke of lightening, but most ascribed the spontaneous organic fire to the existence of an "internal fire."

The case of the poor countess was considered so extraordinary that it was mentioned in the London *Register* of 1763, illustrated at the Academy of Science of France, and reported in a scientific communication by Count Morozzo of the Academy of Arts and Sciences in Turin. What could have been the cause of this autocombustion? From the examination of other victims, it resulted that most had been addicted to alcohol, but in the case of the Countess Bardi, who did not drink, it was supposed that the cause could be traced to the habit of rubbing her body with spirits of camphorated wine before sleeping.

Since Roman times, many believed in the possibility of a sort of autoinflammability, "a marvelous and terrible physical and natural phenomenon that subjects the human machine to spontaneous ignition, without the action of external substances put into combustion."[10] A few centuries later, the abstract theories of romantic-animistic medicine indicated in the phlogiston, a hypothetical element of pure fire believed to exist in combustible bodies, the essential principle that allowed an animal organism to burn: Combustion was due to chemical decomposition and consequent escape of phlogiston. The curious phenomena produced by static electricity, the discovery of oxygen, carbonic acid and hydrogen led many studious men to believe that the human body could burn spontaneously from autocombustion. Therefore, from the Age of Enlightenment to the middle of the nineteenth century, that which for centuries had been considered only a myth became an extraordinary phenomenon of human pathology, worthy of being reported and discussed in serious scientific publications.

In 1773, the Medical Academy of Holland published a dissertation by a certain Doctor Dupont which offered the final proof that a human body could spontaneously catch on fire; this allowed his colleagues to come to the wildest conclusions. Doctor Dupont had discovered during his research that animals, as well as some humans, could emit light and sparks from their eyes: This "fact" led him to the irrefutable conviction that an internal force, a kind of fire which could suddenly burst forth, existed in the human body. His thesis was based on an actual event which had occurred long ago in the sixteenth century: A professor of the University of Pisa was dissecting the body of a young woman whose stomach was strangely dilated; a pupil, venturing too close with a lighted candle, caused a tremendous explosion "with green flames and a horrible smell." The German scientist, J. Heinrich Kopp, described eighteen cases, fourteen of which he had personally witnessed; he took advantage of the occasion to polemicize with another scientist, who conjectured that autocombustion was possible only in females.[11] In an issue of "Judiciary Medicine" published in 1837, F. Pasqualone explained that some people are prone to become victims of spontaneous ignition, especially obese women who consume spirits: As old wood burns more rapidly, elderly women are easier prey to fire. Kopp recounted in detail how fire caused by "live flame, mobile and burning," almost always salvages the hands and feet and leaves "greasy and fetid" residual ashes.[12]

Autoignition was explained as "one of those marvelous occurrences amongst the extraordinary that develop in animal organisms." It "presumes an intimate perversion that our humours sustain" and is caused by electrical sparks that "by physical law decompose water into hydrogen and oxygen that burn with intensity and extraordinary celerity."

Autocombustion became an important literary phenomenon: Emile Zola and Edgar Allan Poe wrote on the subject, exciting the obsessive curiosity of many readers. The best-known book was written by Charles Dickens, who in *Bleak House* describes a case of spontaneous combustion: An old man, Lord Chancelier, addicted to generous daily doses of gin, was found in his cellar, reduced to a sticky, foul-smelling lump of soot.

John Rathbone Oliver describes some of these literary horror stories in an article published in a medical journal in 1936. In his learned dissertation, he evinces that men become "combustible" only when they drink beyond measure and live in disorderly and dirty quarters; if these boozers go near a fire, they can easily go up in flames. This can only happen however to those who drink cheap gin or spirits: No danger exists for those who drink good-quality scotch.[13]

It wasn't long before some charlatans took notice of these facts reported by serious scientific communities. From their practical minds came forth a reasoning beyond argument: If a human being could be combustible, it would be to their advantage to demonstrate that they possessed secret remedies to make a person "incombustible."

Giuseppe Lionet: The "Incombustible" Man

A charlatan named Giuseppe Lionet, a native of Como, arrived in Turin at the end of the eighteenth century declaring himself to be the "real incombustible man." Like every charlatan of any worth, he was preceded by advertisements which claimed that his fame "is well known in Europe and through public documents." He boasted of being able to drink boiling oil, chew melted lead, swallow phosphorus, and, finally, walk into a hot oven holding a rack of lamb and some eggs and not come out until the meat and eggs were well done. He had accomplished this experiment with success, he said, "before the most respectable and erudite medical faculties of Paris, Montpellier, Bordeaux, and Holland."

A serious-minded abbot, Father Giorgio Frollini, professor of philosophy, physics and geometry, teacher at the metropolitan seminary of Turin, assumed the difficult task of revealing the fraud. He had no doubt that some individuals could manifest an exceptional tolerance toward heat and cited as example the case, reported by the Royal Academy of the Sciences, of a Turkish priest who could hold a burning ball in his mouth. At the same time, the abbot was certain that Lionet was not "inferior, in deception and shrewdness, to other quacks." In a booklet titled "On the Presumed Real Incombustible Man," the abbot tenaciously refutes the charlatan's celebrated experiments, demonstrating that his incombustibility was only imaginary, the "artful and fraudulent illusion" of a conjurer. He implacably submitted the poor charlatan to a series of trials, specially designed to prove that he was not insensible: First, the pitiless cleric poured nitric acid on the charlatan's arm, causing a painful burn, and the exasperated charlatan had to admit "not being of iron but a man similar to others." The painful tests came to an end when Lionet was ordered to drink a sip of sulfuric acid and refused to submit to the experiment, saying that he suffered from "some discomfort of health." After this, the abbot was confirmed in his opinion that Lionet was not incombustible and that the "supposed, natural incombustibility, of which he recklessly boasted, by none other is caused than by sleight of hand, practice, and art."[14] Not a word of sympathy transpires from the writings of the meticulous abbot, nor any sign of appreciation for the able conjurer who, like many charlatans who preceded him, risked real lesions with courage and suffering.

A hundred years later, following in the Italian charlatan's wake, Ivanitz Chabert, also defining himself as "the only real incombustible phenomenon," appeared on the London scene. This gentleman really did seem incombustible: In his most celebrated exhibition, he would enter a lighted oven with a tray of raw meat and potatoes; when he came out, the roast was cooked, ready to taste with his guests, and only his cheeks had turned a bright, burning red.

His tricks were considered so exceptional that, according to the newspapers, not even the most illustrious professors of Oxford could discover them. Chabert could swallow phosphorus without damage, put his hands in liquid lead and wash them afterward with corrosive acids, and, for dessert, drink a few spoonfuls of boiling oil. These exhibits, with good cause, made him a phenomenal attraction, and most of the public believed he was endowed with supernatural powers. At last, when Chabert suspected that his secrets were about to be discovered, he emigrated to America, where he dedicated himself to healing; he peddled a cure for rabies, antidotes against poison and other prodigious remedies with the purpose, as he wrote in the *Times*, "of offering great benefits to humanity." Once again the field of medicine had offered a charlatan the chance to make a living.[15]

CHAPTER 12

Mesmerists, Hypnotists, and "Wondrous" Somnambulists

At the beginning of the nineteenth century, along with nostrum mongers who sold their panaceas in the squares and wandering healers who drew the crowds with their histrionic behavior, other quacks appeared who took advantage of the latest discoveries in chemistry, physics, and medical science. In tune with their transformation, these modern charlatans exchanged their fancy clothes for more sober attire and radically modified their behavior: They presented themselves as distinguished professionals, their demeanor serious and reserved; they imitated the gentlemanly gestures of fashionable physicians, receiving clients in their consulting offices with reservedness and doctrinal style. Many used the more convenient and discreet postal correspondence or the silent and diffuse enticement of advertisements in newspapers, which drew the public more efficiently than the racket of drums and trumpets; this circumspection was especially appreciated by aristocrats and the upper-middle classes, who preferred not to expose themselves or ask for advice and remedies in front of everybody, nor find themselves confused amongst the rabble in public places.

In their relations with patients, these "consulting room" charlatans were generally more obliging than physicians. Masters at intertwining truth with falsehood, they created a confusion that was difficult to detect. Their force of conviction was so powerful that by dint of interpreting scientific methods in their own manner, many ended up blindly believing in the virtues of their own remedies and, when needed, chose to cure themselves with their own therapies.

Despite the sensational scientific progression of the century — the discovery of microbes, the revolution created by antisepsis and anesthesia —
most diseases were not yet susceptible to any effective treatment. With
bitter irony, it was said that half of recoveries were due to natural causes,
and the other half came about notwithstanding the physicians' cures. When
not downright harmful, most therapies were totally inefficient; doctors
still prescribed purges, enemas, applications of dry or scarifying cupping
glasses; typhoid fever, cholera, pneumonia and pleurisy, or rheumatism,
were treated with bloodletting.

Meanwhile, new scientific discoveries persuaded people to put all
their hopes in magnetism, hypnotism, electricity and in the mysterious
rays that scientists produced in strange glass tubes after having subjected
them to powerful electrical charges: These manifestations of omnipotent
sciences, still partly inexplicable, created the mirage of omnipotent cures.

Animal Magnetism: Quackery or Science?

A new theory on animal magnetism linked to a universal fluid, proclaimed by an extravagant Viennese physician, opened new horizons in
healing and immediately fascinated the public. The creator of this magnetic force was Franz Anton Mesmer, an intelligent man of undisputed culture, who exploited his personal charm and his gifts of occult hypnotist.

Magnetism was not an entirely new phenomenon: Mesmer and the
magnetizers who, in good or bad faith followed, were the heirs of Paracelsus, the brilliant, revolutionary, sixteenth-century physician and alchemist
who was responsible for the beginning of an irremediable crisis in the
Galeno-Hippocratical medicine of humors. Paracelsus, gifted with a volcanic personality, demonstrated the mysterious therapeutic properties of
the magnet, or loadstone, the incorruptible adamant which would relieve
the physical sufferings of humankind and halt the decline of old age.

A century later, carefully navigating between magic and science, the
Englishman Robert Fludd, an imaginative "doctor of physick," declared
that he could cure any disease with a magnet; the patient had to be placed
in a boreal position during the treatment, for everyone, like the earth, possessed a north and a south pole. His compatriot, the celebrated alchemist
Sir Kenelm Digby, said that the pain of a sword wound could be relieved
through magnetization, simply by rubbing the tip of the offending weapon
with the fingertips.[1]

Other extravagant minds appeared on the scene to suggest that the
magnet's "fluid" could be exploited to create a "sympathetic alphabet"

with which two persons could communicate with each other across a distance of a thousand miles. It was necessary only to transplant a small piece of skin, on which the letters of the alphabet had been written, from the forearm of one man to that of another; when one of the men pricked a letter on the transplanted tissue with a magnetized needle, his distant companion, thanks to the magnetic fluid, would feel a puncture on that same letter. A magnetic telegraph which worked on human skin was an idea that not even the fervid imaginations of quacks had been able to dream up.

In those same years a charlatan named Francesco Bagnone, fervent admirer of the English magnetists, gave exhibitions in many Italian cities. He usually preferred to cure patients of the female gender, touching them with the fluid of his hands, theatrically reinforcing his therapies by making her kneel and pray before a reliquary.

Giuseppe Balsamo, who called himself the Count of Cagliostro, captivated the entire populace of Strasbourg with his incredible healings: He made the lame walk and restored sight to the blind with a touch of his fingers and the sound of his words, an able mixture of fraud and hypnotism. The police had to hold back the throngs who massed in front of his home in Bordeaux. In Saint Petersburg, "the greatest doctor in Europe" offered money to the poor: More hungry than sick, they were rapidly and miraculously cured by the handfuls of rubles that the Count generously bestowed, a spectacular charity that procured him other, more affluent, patients. The accounts of his healings confirm the power of suggestion that his theatrical behavior and hypnotic powers triggered in the frivolous minds of the society of his time. Mystifier of an uncommon breed, Cagliostro was an extraordinary figure who lived in an extraordinary century. His fanciful rascality and the variety of his innumerable hoaxes have justly earned him a place of honor amongst the greatest adventurers, hypnotists, cabalists, and impostors of all times.

Mesmerism

The foremost teacher and inspirer of Mesmer's theory was the Jesuit priest Kircher, who advised patients affected with large hernias to swallow magnetic powder while simultaneously applying iron shavings externally; the magnetic attraction would immediately cause the herniated viscera to reenter. Mesmer, at the beginning of his career, also experimented with the therapeutic action of magnetized metal plaques, placing them over aching parts, but soon he realized that he could provoke the same effects simply by transmitting the magnetic fluid from his hands to the body of his patient.

Mesmer's theory on the existence of a universal fluid was made public in Vienna; in a lengthy dissertation, he explained the reciprocal influence of the planets on humankind, a veritable celestial-animal magnetism which in a short while procured resounding success for its inventor. After moving to Paris, in the course of memorable exhibitions, he provoked uncontrollable phenomena of collective suggestion and miraculous healings with the sort of behavior that had little of the physician and much of the charlatan of a very rare species. A refined speaker, of handsome appearance, dressed in lilac satin adorned with fine lace, Mesmer possessed all the hypnotic gifts that were necessary to exert, especially on the female gender, an irresistible fascination. His patients sat trustfully around a large magnetic tub; each of them was connected to an iron bar that transmitted the fluid which issued from bottles of magnetized water. The clients held each others' hands, their knees in tight contact to better transmit the mysterious fluid.

The ambiance was luxurious: From vast adjacent parlors the sound of harps could be heard, and perfumes and vapors of incense wafted on the air while the young and handsome assistants of the maestro distributed the animal fluid, practicing light massages on various parts of the body, including sensual "pressures" on the breasts of the ladies, that "sweet and fervid prey" that thronged to the sessions.[2] Soon the participants began to writhe with convulsions; the women cried and tore their hair, everyone screamed and sobbed. Only when Mesmer appeared, and solemnly touched them with his magic wand did the delirium cease. The results of these sessions were incredible, and soon the fame of the Viennese doctor spread all over Europe.

Even though Mesmer enjoyed the public's favor and the protection of the aristocrats and the royal court, the academic faculty strongly resisted mesmerism. A commission of illustrious experts from the prestigious Academy of Sciences, in which Benjamin Franklin participated, decreed that magnetic animal magnetism was only a phenomenon of crooked and dangerous suggestion; Mesmer was ordered to stop his exhibitions.

His luck began to run out from that moment on; even his most enthusiastic advocates, reunited in the Society of Harmony, began to doubt the reliability of the hypnotist's claims, for he refused to reveal the secret of his universal fluid. In a few years, partly because of the upheavals brought on by the French Revolution, the famous charlatan-physician lost all his prestige. The remaining years of his life were spent wandering about Europe, until he died, almost entirely forgotten.

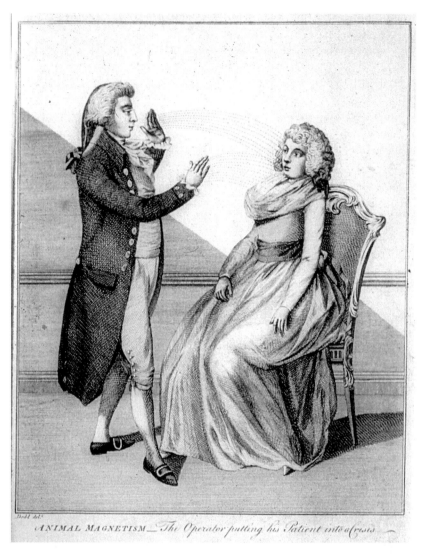

ANIMAL MAGNETISM.—The Operator putting his Patient into a Crisis.—

A follower of Mesmer uses his magnetic fluid to induce a trance in a lady. Engraving by Dodd (1774). U.S. National Library of Medicine, Bethesda, MD.

Nonetheless, animal magnetism had gained such popularity with the public that Mesmerian sessions continued for the whole of the nineteenth century, encouraging numerous followers that were even more extravagant than their famous teacher. Several medical treatises explained magnetism. T. Elton, in 1865, described a mesmeric session: The patient sat on an armchair while the hypnotist, after ordering the patient to sleep, transmitted the fluid by making several passes with his hands in front of the patient's eyes, head and shoulders.[3]

Legions of medical and nonmedical quacks, either for lucre or for exhibitionism, claimed to possess Mesmer's gifts and the means to connect their patients to cosmic emissions, although the only connection that was usually made was with their own pocketbooks. Mesmerism seemed to be entirely in the hands of visionaries and charlatans in bad faith; their insane pronouncements passed every rational limit; they not only claimed that they could cure every disease but also that any ignorant person, charged with magnetic fluid, could be made to discuss philosophical arguments, speak strange foreign tongues, and absorb the learning in books, merely by holding them open on their knees.

Requests for licensed physicians that would assist mesmerists and their somnambulists appeared in city newspapers: "Magnetizing" clinics could obtain authorization only if a physician took responsibility for the cure. In the principle Italian cities, these so-called magnetizing clinics enlisted clairvoyant somnambulists who were supposed to diagnose the illness and give a prescription for its treatment during a trance. Clients who were unable to attend in person had only to send in a list of symptoms, "enclosing a lock of hair and five lira."[4]

The somnambulists either gave medical diagnoses or acted as simple fortunetellers. In Treviso, a magnetizer exhibited a somnambulist, actually his own wife, who sat in an armchair in the middle of the square, pretentiously dressed with a fancy little cape decorated with lace, and a large hat with feathers; she held a satin umbrella and wore a long chain of fake gold around her neck and ten shiny rings on her right hand. After covering her with a black veil, the mesmerist announced to the public assembled in the square the wonderful talents of "this phenomenon, for she was born a seventh-month baby," a creature blessed by fortune for having been born two months early. Divination was not a difficult task: Often the somnambulist was able to see through a thin opening cut in the large black veil that covered her face, or else her husband, talking in a jargon incomprehensible to others, enabled her to guess extraordinary things about each client.

In a sensational trial, celebrated in Turin, the defendant was a self-styled "Professor" Filippa, a magnetizer who, aided by a medical accomplice, offered "magnetical consultations for every sort of disease and curiosity." Filippa used a somnambulist who gave diagnoses and dispensed unfailing treatments while in a trance. The "Criminal Review," which published the trial, commented: "The title of Professor" [with which Filippa had adorned his name] "by now in common usage, has a meaning that is so widespread, so elastic, that it embraces the very infinite mercy of God."[5]

Public manifestations of magnetism gave rise to confused and opposing interpretations; many clerics judged them as supernatural events organized by the devil himself; most physicians believed that they were instances of hypnotic trance; skeptics, who were in the majority, were convinced that they were due to the theatrical ability of the charlatans, aided by complaisant accomplices. Toward the end of the century, the Royal Academy of Medicine requested that public displays of hypnotism be forbidden because they provoked perturbation of mental faculties.

Animal magnetism, although destined to be banished to the museum of frauds, if nothing else had the merit of improving the relationship between doctor and patient and foreshadowed the possibility of using methods of therapy directed to the mind. A naturalist who participated in the commission which condemned Mesmer did not concur with the other scientists; he too admitted that animal magnetism did not exist, but he claimed that it was impossible to discount the mysterious but undeniable phenomenon of imagination which, at least temporarily, had demonstrated its ability to produce some relief, if not complete healing.

Franco Voltaggio more recently wrote, "Without doubt, science has taken advantage of the vast movement born of the naive and often mistaken conceptions of animal magnetism"; later it will find "not only scientific expression in psychoanalytical transfer but also in homeopathy, and in many other non-orthodox methods of cure it will be the secret of success for other softer, more natural, more spiritual medicines."[6]

Charlatans: "Loathsome Leprosy That Infects and Assails All of Society"

This dramatic declaration was written in the middle of the nineteenth century by Giuseppe Berruti, a doctor and brilliant journalist, the sworn enemy of every kind of quackery, which he defined as "mythical might, monster, extraordinary and marvelous power, desire cast between ignorance and fanaticism, strength of soothsayers, of somnambulists, of thaumaturges and empirics, from whom the poor, desperate, gullible, and ignorant people are unable to flee." Not only did Berruti oppose those who were charlatans by trade; anyone who stepped outside the canons of official medicine was a charlatan, and little did it matter if he was a licensed physician or an ignoramus, for, "unfortunately, even amongst doctors, to our disgrace many are unable to elude this imaginary occult power."[7] From his own point of view, he was not entirely wrong; the number of doctors who "sacrificed themselves on the altar of their purses" by transforming themselves into charlatans continuously increased. In 1922 Andrea Corsini wrote of a physician, a certain Dr. Groppi, who, while in Padua, was attracted by a charlatan selling plasters and other miraculous remedies in Piazza delle Erbe. At a certain point, the charlatan noticed the doctor's presence and jumped down from his platform to ask him for an appointment, which the doctor, to avoid embarrassment, readily gave him. When the charlatan arrived at his studio, Dr. Groppi realized that the man was a former companion at the university, the brightest in the class; for eight years, he had earned only a pittance as a country doctor and had decided to become a quack; since then, practicing in the public squares, he had earned enough money to be able to retire.[8]

A well-known doctor wrote at the beginning of the twentieth century, "Tomorrow, if any type of quack should arrive in Rome, Chicago, or Peking preceded by colossal posters or by an avalanche of many published pages which state that without any doubt he can recognize and can cure any sort of tumor, one would be able to assist at a most interesting scene … and would see, hastening in admirable promiscuity with the most illiterate boors, not only illustrious men of letters, subtle politicians and philosophers as profound as the ocean, but most amazing of all, one would discover, confused in the crowd's midst, fearful of being exposed, even some physician who has definitely lost faith in his own art."[9]

Medical advertisements in newspapers became a powerful aid to quackery: Not by chance did Mark Twain warn his readers to take care before blindly following medical precepts that could be read in the press: They could die because of a misprint.

As the process of commercialization of medicine went on apace, the first pharmaceutical companies, backed by a shameless publicity, flooded the market with products of all kinds, for the most part absolutely useless. Often the vilest proceedings and the basest compromises were hidden beneath a veneer of seeming honesty; as in our own times, pharmaceutical advertisements were simplified and presented as scientific information.

The cleverest charlatans relied on the discoveries of Pasteur or of some other illustrious scientist to propagandize their new theories; they presented therapeutic methods that implied the harnessing of vital forces of nature. Recently discovered roentgen rays and mysterious hypnotic fluids produced a confused tangle in the minds of many people, even amongst the most cultured; some superior minds, including the celebrated scientist Crookes, discoverer of the radiations that bear his name, blindly believed in spiritism, accepting it as being caused by a mysterious, powerful fluid. It was a time in which inspired healers, skillful defrauders of simpletons, were appearing all over Europe.

While fashionable healers, serious and self-possessed, received their clients with grave professorial style, tooth drawers, nostrum mongers, quack doctors, jesters and players with small caravans could still be met in the countryside or village fairs. Most were bizarre and colorful figures who thrilled and amused the public with ostentatious pomp, irresistible loquacity and every type of ruse.

The writer Renato Fucini left colorful accounts and indelible impressions of Tofani and Bennati, two ingenious artists who "practiced their miraculous art in the squares, standing on a wagon or on the roof of a carriage." Here is Tofani, "a handsome male, strong, with flowing and curly hair ... pleasing voice, fluid speech, flashing eyes, sly and kind smile alternated with a wild beast's glare." During the prologue of his declamation, the charlatan makes a display of his medical knowledge, reminiscing about his miraculous healings, continuously leafing through a "great huge book" which contains all the testimonials granted to him by celebrities all over the world. The silent and admiring crowd, the writer recounts, parted to reveal "gaping mouths, withered limbs, scrofulous children, mugs gnawed by lupus, rheumy eyes": samples of distress, inhabitants of a poor and humble Italy to which Tofani gave temporary hope in exchange for a few small coins.

The other charlatan, Bennati, practiced his art in a "show of pageantry with which he noisily presented himself in the squares." Fucini describes his triumphal entrance into Empoli, a large town in Tuscany: "[A]round nine on Thursday morning a shrill blare of trumpets was heard and soon after, relays on horseback appeared, in elegant liveries of brilliant colors. At a well calculated distance from the horsemen traveled the great catafalque of the majestic carriage, pulled by four horses, on which he, Bennati, stood on his feet with Olympian calm, his breast overloaded with medals, surrounded by a thick group of his accomplices, male and female, dressed as negroes, as red skinned Americans, as near-naked cannibals from Oceania, and disguised in various styles that have never existed under the mantle of the sun, who gesticulated and talked to the diabolic sound of an infernal orchestra."

Almost the entire population of Empoli hastened to see Bennati's show; the thaumaturge did not disappoint them; from his carriage, he cast coins of various denominations which the frenzied crowd struggled to gather up. Afterwards, as the square settled into utter silence, "he never ceased pulling teeth, cutting veins, binding wounds, straightening backbones and crooked legs, healing the gnawings of lupus, phagedenic ulcers and lethal cancers," all this accompanied by the ever more deafening din of music. While Bennati operated, "three or four characters, hanging from the carriage, tirelessly peddled powders, liquids, infallible prescriptions, orthopaedical instruments, unguents and concoctions of every kind. In this way, the money, the coins that he had sowed a brief time before, after a short pause returned to his pockets." It is understandable that Fucini, the son of a country doctor, considered charlatans no more than "leftovers from barbarism ... the ensigns of antiscience, the obstructers of medical progress, the most vulgar of rabble-rousing demagogues."[10]

The Italian charlatans' custom of accompanying themselves with large traveling companies created the fashion for this kind of trade throughout the world; these same attractions, these same mass spectacles, were repeated and perfected with local variations everywhere. Troupes of players traveled about the United States, the head quack combining histrionic gestures with the nonsense of a circus performer and often accompanied by a tribe of Native Americans who rode on wild horses and by a company of players and singers. Indian dances were performed to the tumult of drums, and afterwards some Negroes entertained the spectators with their tomfoolery. The very same ostentatious acts that companies of charlatans had performed in Italy for centuries were being repeated in a faraway country.

The Autobiography of a Socialist Charlatan

In the dark years of the last world war, Arturo Frizzi, a quack from Mantova who had practiced his trade from the end of the nineteenth century right up to World War I, died, blind and forgotten. He had been an able swindler, one that would not have cut a poor figure in the colorful gallery of popular quacks that Tomaso Garzoni had described with such incisiveness four centuries earlier.

Frizzi saw no contradiction in mingling together good-natured frauds, cynicism, bad faith and his personal convictions that extolled social liberty: "I am socialist and communist," he confessed in a ponderous autobiography, "for I believe it is just that to every living person at every instant be given the means to obtain his need." The satisfaction that this extravagant man felt whenever he was able to dupe someone was worth more than the little money he scraped together to feed himself.

Political author and modest editor, in 1912 he published a book, *The Charlatan*, that has become a classic in the literature on quackery. In it he recounts his real life experiences during a period of rapid social, cultural and economic changes.[11]

In reality, his activities in the field of medicine were superficial, and his vaunted knowledge of herbal remedies was quite cursory. A companion of like kind, a certain Ferdinando Marchionni, owned a liquor and coffee shop in Pisa; although Marchionni was endowed with "exceptional shrewdness," as Frizzi writes, "he was soon left without coffee or liquor, and without money because of his gold heart." Both of them received a sudden "dentistic" inspiration after they had observed the fortune of a real tooth drawer, a charlatan who was so rich that he entered the city "mounted on an elegant carriage, with four splendid horses, servants in livery and eight musicians." Trusting that they too would make money by imitating this fortunate rival, the two arrived in the large market square of Pisa and quickly set up a table, "covering it with a beautiful damask carpet belonging to Marchionni." Then they persuaded a shop owner to lend them a "tray with two beautiful branched candelabra with four lighted candles, a bottle of water, two small glasses," and even a crucifix. A flashy and pompous show reminiscent of the duel that the Unknown Cavalier organized in the mid-eighteenth century against his rival, the Cosmopolitan.

Frizzi explained that timing is the most important element in a quack's profession. He must recognize the exact moment in which to offer his merchandise, but, like a virgin, he has to be very cautious before "opening his bag; … if she waits too long, she becomes an old maid, if she anticipates, she becomes the victim of a catastrophe."

The secret of the show was entrusted to some mysterious black pills, manufactured by the famous pharmaceutical company Erba of Milan, which the two kept locked in a small box. The pills were actually balls of excrement "sowed by sheep as they grazed," with a "pit" of putrid cheese full of worms which the two accomplices had put inside each one. Frizzi, "whom mother nature had furnished with two iron lungs and a glibness of tongue that would be the envy of any lawyer," began to declaim: "Gentlemen! Here is the beneficial vegetable pill which will make toothache disappear and kill the horrible cavity."

When the first spectator had taken a pill from its wrapper and pressed it onto his aching tooth, Frizzi then put the pill on the tray and showed "the terrible insect" to all those present: It was none other than a worm taken from the rotting cheese. After this incontrovertible demonstration, the astonished onlookers were convinced, and the poor patient, influenced "by the crowd that contemplated him, the charlatan that magnetized him by staring in his eyes, swore before the crucifix that the pill had removed all his pain." In the blink of an eye, all the pills were sold, with the immense satisfaction and gain of the two merry frauds.

Frizzi and his companion did not invent the jolly practical joke based on dental worms. In the year A.D. 162, the famous Roman physician Galen, while strolling through a market, noticed a quack surrounded by a group of simpletons. "I have met Galen," the man cried, "who taught me everything he knows. Here is a remedy for the teeth." The charlatan had prepared little balls of tar; setting one alight, he held it in front of the patient's face so that the smoke kept the man from opening his eyes; then he quickly put a worm from a little jar into the man's mouth and pretended to pull it out. The bystanders offered him all the money they had, but at this point Galen suddenly presented himself to the crowd, saying, "I am Galen and he is a fraud," and immediately had the man apprehended and whipped.[12]

Just like the nostrum mongers who were also comic actors, Frizzi and his companion continued a popular art form that the writer Ardengo Soffici described with nostalgia, remembering the years of his youth and the fairy-tale impression that he received "in the fairs amongst the countless, colorful stalls, and the fanfare and shouts of mountebanks and charlatans who delighted the crowd pressed close around and flooding the rest of the square, in a high din of cries and trumpets."[13]

Enticing Instruments and Mysterious Rays

The discoveries of bacteria, vaccines, anesthesia and antisepsis restored lost social prestige to the practice of medicine; after these technical and scientific revolutions it would have been logical to believe that the days of quackery were over and that the triumph of orthodox medicine would finally lop off the protean Hydra's head, but these very same novelties of modern technology offered charlatans alternate means, both powerful and alluring. Italian charlatans, less creative in these new fields, now concentrated on imitating and propagandizing the complicated contrivances invented and sold for the most part in Anglo-Saxon countries.

Instruments became the greatest innovation of nineteenth-century quackery: electric corsets, irradiating batteries, fake rays. The most disparate contraptions could cure all ills, restore lost vigor, procure youth and beauty. Machines of every sort were produced, mechanical devices designed to prevent masturbation or enlarge the breasts by means of a suction pump; hydraulic contrivances to squeeze pimples or increase the pressure in enema pumps. A proliferation of gadgets appeared that were designed to exploit electricity, the most fascinating and exalting of all the prodigies which fascinated the public, a fascination that was the determinant for a profitable commercial activity: the sale of electrical instruments alleged to aid the recovery of lost health.

A so-called Academy of Electricity declared in the newspapers that "no pain, no weakness, can resist electricity, which has the power to saturate the nerves with electrical vitality and spread it to every organ and tissue of the body, bestowing health, strength, and vigor!" Even accredited academic circles accepted the idea that many therapies, such as purges and sulfur, had an effect on the organism due to their positive or negative electrical charges. Some physicians even presented electrical apparatuses to scientific academies, promising to restore sight to the blind and hearing to the deaf; it was difficult to distinguish inventors in good faith from charlatans.

Countless metal utensils associated with electrical current were advertised for years by foreign quacks and later imported and acclaimed in Italy. An "English Electrical Company" with considerable hyperbole offered a simple light bulb attached to a battery; used at least three times a day, it would reduce the weakness of vision "brought on by age or other excesses." Later, electricity would be used for opposite purposes: The number of people who were convinced that electricity was necessary to expel a disease dwindled in respect to those who recommended it as a remedy to restore lost vital forces.[14]

A foreign name and provenance were essential for every device: a cunning merchant flooded the newspapers with ads claiming that some medical consultants received patients in Milan free of charge, even on Sundays, so that they could try "Electro-Vigor," an electric belt that would "increase resistance and strength in the body tenfold, an indispensable instrument for men who have now lost every ambition and all hope due to premature aging. For these cases, salvation is in electricity." The same company offered five thousand lira for every disease that could not be cured with their instruments, which "cause the admiration of electricians, as they dispose of the most potent curative force that has ever been known." A few years later, *Policlinico*, the most reliable and widely circulated Italian medical journal, announced that the company that produced Electro-Vigor, had been strictly proscribed from selling the belt after a sensational trial in Paris. But quacks quickly found other expedients: Other advertisements in Italian newspapers propagandized new electrical instruments; this time it was guaranteed that electricity was furnished by dry batteries.

For a time, improvised Italian quacks offered "mechanical vibrators." These instruments had a multiplying mechanism that was set in motion manually with a handle and were meant to cure every ailing part of the body with their rapid vibrations: "a scientific device, perfect in its vibrating massage, capable of producing ten thousand vibrations of adjustable intensity a minute; it is provided with twelve shakers or tremblers of various consistency and form, adaptable according to the parts of the body and different infirmities."[15] The fiendish "tremblers" were implements of various forms that were introduced into the mouth to cure hair loss, migraine headaches and rheumatism, or into the anus to treat hemorrhoids, nocturnal enuresis, and so on. Fortunately they did not have much success, even if the advertisements stated that they had been adopted by many "clinics and institutes of the kingdom."

Once X rays had been discovered, not much time passed before someone, going backward in the alphabet, announced the discovery of "V" rays: reddish rays that emanated even from the eyes of certain people. These rays too could pass through objects and leave an image on film and thereby investigate the inner body. In the early years, medical X-ray machines operated in the dark, accompanied by a flashing of sparks. Some quacks or even doctors with few scruples were discovered during consultation with fake machines that had no radiating tube but a multitude of colored lights. The patient sat dumbfounded, terrified, awaiting with dread the diagnosis of his disease, surrounded by glittering lights and the crackling of sparks, artfully contrived with powerful electrical discharges.

For many years after the Curies' sensational discoveries it was believed advisable to drink radioactive solutions as a cure for a multitude of diseases, with no thought of the potential hidden dangers. Luckily, many of these mixtures either did not contain the slightest radiant power, or else the radioactive content was so low that it did not cause much damage. Most famous spa waters were advertised as being radioactive; an immersion in a tub or a half glass of radioactive water drunk every morning was supposed to be enough to procure beneficial effects for both adults and children.

Toward the end of the 1920s, trusting multitudes traveled to a village in Bohemia where Valentin Zileis offered treatments with electricity and radium. All the inhabitants of the town were involved in the business of hosting thousands of patients, naturally for a fee. After waiting long hours in the "Praeparatorium," the patients entered the "Mysterium," a room whose walls were decorated with paintings of serpents; a skeleton, illuminated with red lights, hung from the center of the ceiling. When they were sufficiently overwhelmed, the quack-magician came onto the scene and made rapid passages with his wand over their bodies, guessing the nature of their illnesses by the intensity of the flashes that came from his marvelous instrument. Once the diagnostic procedure was over, the group of patients was treated collectively with blinding flashes of lightening produced by an electrical contraption, followed by a treatment with high-frequency X rays for one or two minutes, "intensified by radium"; finally they were exposed to rays from a helium lamp. This infernal shower of lights and radiation repaid its inventor nicely: Each day, the two thousand patients treated in this manner filled his pockets with five or six thousand marks![16]

Electricity was elected to cure tuberculosis, the most dreaded disease of the nineteenth century. The proposed official cures, besides being useless, were often dangerous: In 1843 a famous clinician of the University of Paris wrote a treatise, later translated for Italian universities: "[I]f the skin is hot, or there is fever, or hemoptysis, then blood should be let. Under the influence of sanguineous emissions, it can often be seen that the symptoms cease." He recommended other useful remedies: cauterization under the collarbone, broths made from breast of veal, or tortoise, snails and frogs, and cauteries on the chest to facilitate expectoration.

The painful history of tuberculosis is an example of how medical knowledge can retrogress instead of progressing. At the end of the fifteenth century, Gerolamo Fracastoro, with amazing intuition, suggested the presence of "seminaria," little creatures that he believed responsible for the transmission of the disease, even if at that time he had no way to see them with a microscope. Accordingly, he advised burning all infected utensils and clothes, which he called "fomites," or receptacles for these little creatures.

Contagion, which was oddly denied and even derided by many scientific luminaries right in the midst of a century that was otherwise full of important discoveries, was the cause of an infinite number of disasters. René-Théophile-Hyacinthe Laënnec, inventor of the stethoscope, which paved the way for clinical examination of the lungs and heart, declared that "tuberculosis was contagious only in the eyes of the world"; a French colleague curiously affirmed that it was contagious "only in Spain."

In the midst all these mistakes, uncertainties and blunders of medical science, fraud and extravagant errors became probable and frequent. At the end of the eighteenth century, the English physician Thomas Beddoes, founder of the Pneumatic Institute for the study of gas, or "artificial air," concluded that the breath of large animals could be beneficial to the lungs of consumptives, either because they withdrew oxygen from the air, or because they added alkaline exhalations. The doctor had the peculiar habit of taking a cow with him on his rounds, prescribing that some of these gentle but cumbersome beasts be put in the rooms around the beds of his poor patients, with results that can be easily imagined.[17]

A marine climate was believed to have a favorable effect on several forms of tuberculosis. Some doctors believed that the benefits were not due to the sea breezes, but to the rolling of a ship or even to sea sickness; they pointed out the fact that many patients returned cured from a lengthy sea voyage. In 1843 the official organ of the Florentine Medical Society printed the opinions of celebrated English and French academics, who thought that it could be extremely beneficial to have the patient sway back and forth on a swing for long hours, preferably in the vicinity of a beach, or ride on long trips in an open carriage. A more unassuming doctor from Trento declared that he had obtained good results simply by giving large doses of strong wine to consumptives, after they had copiously perspired during tiring physical exercises.[18]

Error, ignorance, pedantry: All are present in the advice of an Italian physician who prescribed for Paganini, sapped by tuberculosis, the cure of Le Roy, a fashionable French charlatan who adorned himself with the title of "Consulting Surgeon." According to Le Roy's theory, most consumptives were "putridfermented," and their disease could be overcome only by drastic purging. "The intestine," he declared, "is like a furnace which is not consumed, but preserved, by removing the rust." If the purge did not have the desired effect, the dose was increased, enough to cause twelve discharges a day. The purging and emollient brew, a deadly bomb made of jalap, senna, and scammony, was Le Roy's decisive contribution to the murder of the greatest violinist of all times. Paganini, influenced by Le Roy's conceits, upheld the effectiveness of the cure, even going as far as to declare that the purge had finally unmasked medical impotence. But not much time passed before the ghostly figure of the incomparable artist was taken from this life by an irrepressible hemoptysis.

CHAPTER 13

Yearned-For,
Eternal Youth

Was the "precious liquor" distilled by the Cistercian monk Don Silvio Boccone a cleverly invented swindle or the result of an ingenuous illusion? In a long letter addressed to "The Illustrious Sir Thomas Vuilloughy, Baronet of London," published in Boccone's *Museum of Physik and Experiences of Natural Observations*, the learned naturalist swears that "by his own experience" this fragrant liquor "was conserved uncorrupted for many Hundreds of years, in a Glass Urn, in which some Ashes and several bones of a Cadaver were enclosed, and deposited."

A "Precious Liquor" Obtained by
a Gruesome Experiment

In the year 1680, in a grave near the canonical grounds of the Old City of Malta, some stone cutters found a glass urn containing a liquid in which a kind of shiny yellow dust floated. Unfortunately, the urn was broken by the "insolence of the greedy Workers, who thought they had found gold." All the inhabitants of Malta were soon possessed by a desire to know what kind of "Balsamic Liquor could this have been that had conserved its enchanting, and uncorrupted fragrance after a series of Hundreds of years?" Surely it was an imperishable liquor that could preserve youth, an "Artificial liquor, and Balsamic" exuded by a cadaver and afterward prepared with special resins, for it was too plentiful to be "the humour collected from the eyes, or from the tears of Relatives." Don Silvio, whose obvious intent was to attract the English nobleman's curiosity and sell him the precious liquor dearly, describes how he was able to recreate this very same liquor. In order to prove the scientific seriousness of his experiment, he tells of his encounters with a certain erudite Melchiorre Sebizio, expert in cadavers, author of a learned "disputation" on the "Conditura aut Balsamatione Cadaverum Humanorum." Their gruesome experiment on the hand and foot of a woman's corpse began in Padua. The piteous remains were first treated with "Varnish of Wax and Terebinth to evacuate the humidity within as is the style of Shoemakers." Boccone and Sebizo then placed the parts in a bath of spirits of wine, myrrh, and aloe for a length of time and afterward dried them at the "heat of digestion." At last, a liquid, the arcane essence that would preserve eternal youth, seeped from a hole in the bottom of the urn.[1]

We do not know if this public letter ever had a response or if the young Englishman was convinced enough to buy Don Silvio's "Incorruptible Liquor." We can only accompany with our imagination the courier as he arrives in London after an exhausting trip over land and sea and delivers into the baronet's hands the miraculous elixir, enclosed in a fragile phial of Venetian glass, along with the monk's prescription. The nobleman would have proudly shown the precious liquor to his friends and then replaced it carefully in its casket, saving it to be sipped slowly in a silver cup during the damp and silent London evenings. If he did not die of an infection contracted from this concentrate of disgusting matter, the noble Thomas Vuilloughy, artfully influenced by the words of the astute Sicilian naturalist, would have probably experienced an indescribable sensation of reinvigoration and gained an invaluable temporary relief from his ailments.

The legendary Fountain of Youth, which Ponce de Leon hoped to find in the West Indies and present as his finest gift to the king of Spain, inspired Cranach's painting of a magic pool where hairless old women, bent with age, immerse themselves in the gushing water and rise, after the salutary bath, fresh and seductive, with smooth pink skin and long black hair. Utopia does not belong to any special era, and over the centuries, the most fertile domain for deceitful fantasies has been man's aspiration to push forward the limit established by our biological lifespan.

Leonardo Fioravanti, who knew the art of fraud well, wrote in one of his books: "[M]an will adapt himself to anything in order to lengthen his life ... and this is a field of human thought where much superstition and much quackery can be found."[2] The prince of charlatans once again was right: Each period has its secret remedies, each society, each generation has experimented with every means to make life last longer.

In Chinese medicine, there are a thousand names of elixirs that purport to grant immortality, made from all kinds of substances: herbs, mercury, urine. The Egyptians not only purged themselves and induced vomiting, but continuously subjected the anus to fumigation, for it was considered the bastion against physical decadence due to age.

When the "human tree begins to wither from deficiency of humor," the philosopher Marsilio Ficino recommended eating myrobalan, a kind of plum believed to grow only in Arabia, but after the age of seventy, "nothing is better than sucking milk from a buxom young girl, when the moon is waxing; and straight away eat a little powder of fennel confectioned with sugar. And if need be, drink human blood." The pursuit of eternal life led to the unedifying episode of a physician who proposed "revitalizing" Pope Innocent VII with a transfusion of blood taken from three ten-year-old boys, who offered themselves for a pathetic recompense. The poor children died after a copious bloodletting, and the physician fled precipitously. The story may have been an invention, circulated to discredit the doctor, who was a Jew.

Advice given to pontiffs to help them prolong their lives was often inauspicious: At the end of the fifteenth century, Gabriele Zerbi dedicated a treaty to Innocent VIII, in which he compared "cold old age" to winter, and the decrepitude of the old man to the inevitable wear and tear of a body that has been used for too long and needs to be warmed by a vital energy. His concepts were more theoretical than practical, for the pope died soon afterward. Some gerontocomedies refuse to disappear: From King David to Mao Tse Tung, many venerable old men continued to believe that it is possible to regain the intense sensations of lost youth by lying with very young girls.

Skeptical and sarcastic as always, Scipione Mercuri warned readers to stay away from charlatans who practiced magic arts and promised that their methods would help regain health, youth and beauty; they used "magic arts such as iron tempered in many sauces, ... thread spun by a virgin girl, a wolf's tail, a deer's brain, a toad's stump and fox's hair and mule's hoof ... with many other foolish things that infect the world." Mercuri expressed his annoyance with those who fear death "with constant sighing but with hot tears and afflicted moans, as if death were not a natural destiny for all." He admonished them "For those who find death grievous, every moment is dead."[3]

From the Middle Ages, the Philosopher's Stone was believed to represent the universal panacea; the man who found this stone would not only be able to convert base metals into gold, but would also be able to guarantee youth, beauty and wealth. For centuries, the stone aroused astonishing fantasies and expectations, some expressed in genuine good faith, some invented with shameless duplicity. The art of alchemy captivated many noble spirits and fueled the optimistic hopes of multitudes. Even Roger Bacon firmly believed in the Philosopher's Stone and spent many hours in its quest. During the sixteenth and seventeenth centuries, thousands of researchers, as enthusiastic as they were unlucky, passed their time arduously searching for the Philosopher's Stone: Amongst these were many callous frauds. Some swore that they had seen it, similar to a ruby, "transparent and fragile as glass," and that they had verified its magic properties; others vowed that they had produced it in their laboratories. It was sufficient to dissolve a grain of the stone in white wine and drink the potion in a silver cup after midnight to prolong life.

Famous alchemists, who claimed to possess the secrets necessary to make the Philosopher's Stone, found a favorable reception at the courts of the most important kings and princes of Europe; after a short time, those bereft of sufficient cunning ended up in prison. Not everyone allowed himself to be duped: The poet and alchemist Augurello da Padova went to Pope Leo X in 1441, swearing that he possessed the stone and could transmute base metal into gold. The pontiff listened to him benevolently and offered him the most appropriate gift: an empty purse in which to put the gold.[4]

Pietro d'Apone from Padua, who lived at the beginning of the fourteenth century, was a medical quack gifted in astronomy and alchemy; he declared that he owned seven jars with seven diabolical spirits who came from seven infernal regions. By opening one of these jars at will, he could uncover the secret of every art. Of the seven, the spirit who dispensed immortality was the one most requested.

Juleps, Electuaries, Quintessences, and Herbolates

A great change occurred when Paracelsus urged physicians to abandon the ancient Galenic therapies of juleps, electuaries, and ground pearls and dedicate their time to separating and recombining the constituent parts of primitive elements until they found the quintessence, the indispensable principle necessary to "create arcanums and oppose them to the diseases," a fanciful idea that at least had the merit of stimulating research for the first chemical remedies. Erasmus of Rotterdam, a great humanist and a man of learning, fell into the trap himself, affirming that this quintessence "is not a fable ... for man rejuvenates and testimony is not lacking."

Leonardo Fioravanti upheld that the only true "quinta essentia" was his own secret, prepared with a mixture of various vegetable and animal substances, an elixir that should be drunk slowly, so effective that it would resuscitate the dying. The powerful effect of his elixir was due mostly to the corroborating action of a strong distilled wine; for this reason Fioravanti made fun of those doctors who uselessly prescribed sweet decoctions and quintessences in syrup.[5]

The so-called herbolates, the mixtures of plants that charlatans offered, were more effective, or at least, inoffensive. The charlatan Antonio Faentino, protégé of Duke Alfonso of Ferrara, swore that he had "conserved many gentlemen who deserved to be immortal in prosperous good health and long life." He mentions the "brothers of the illustrious House of Este and many others too numerous to name…, who, thanks to his *Elettuario Vitae*, had happily passed their eightieth year." Unfortunately these eminent gentlemen had not followed his instructions exactly, otherwise they would still be alive, for his electuary "would have been sufficient to make them perpetual and immortal."[6]

Sebastiano Benelli, a fanciful, eighteenth century herbalist who called himself professor "chemist," described the occult properties of galega, or goat's rue, in a small book titled *The Terror of Death*. An Egyptian doctor, encountered on the island of Malta, confessed that by virtue of this portentous herb he had reached the respectable age of 184 years, and his father, who looked younger than the son, had passed 200.[7]

Even if they were tepidly credulous, people eyed these portentous secrets with a certain skepticism; in a part of their being they were amused, not at the charlatans, but at their own absurd hope. In the eighteenth century, the artist Mitelli engraved a scene that could have been suitable for a quack's calling card: A patient half lifts himself out of bed to blow in the Grim Reaper's face. The caption reads: "The unerring secret to never die: when death comes to take you, straight away blow in his face, but be sure never to stop, for when you stop, you are dead"—a marvelous discovery, easy and infallible.

With the auspices of science, the mirage of a remedy that would halt the inexorable passage of time seemed near at hand; many doctors even outstripped quacks with their fantasy. Metchnikoff, a Russian researcher gifted with a volcanic mind, winner of the Nobel prize in 1908, believed that he had discovered the causes of old age in hydrogenated substances that were produced in stasis and fermentation of the colon. His solution was of astounding simplicity: All that was necessary to add years to one's life was to eat huge quantities of yogurt like the Bulgarian peasants did. Lured by the temptation to find a quick solution to a problem, Metchnikoff had made one of the most frequent errors in medicine by arbitrarily associating two events—longevity and the abundant ingestion of yogurt—convincing himself that the two were in some way connected.

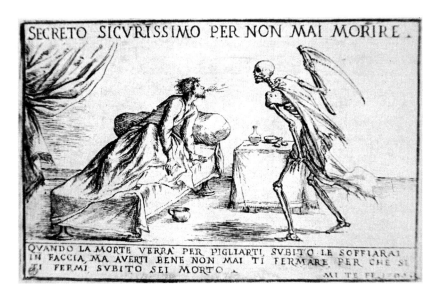

A Sure Secret Never to Die. *"As long as the patient can stil blow in the face of the Grim Reaper, he will not die."* Satirical engraving by Giuseppe Mitelli (1706). Biblioteca Nazionale Centrale, Firenze.

Other physicians accepted the idea of a "homicidal colon" and adhered to the Russian scientist's sensational revelation without a prolonged phase of experiment. Victor Pauchet, professor of clinical medicine, advised young men who were about to get married to discreetly investigate their future bride's intestinal functioning. If a dangerous intestinal stasis was suspected, he counseled them to procrastinate or even to find an excuse to cancel the wedding.[8] In the 1930s, the respected English surgeon Sir Arbunothnot Lane intervened more drastically, cutting out large sections or even the entire intestine if he believed that it was obstructed by adhesions which might favor a highly dangerous fermentation; these interventions, besides being useless, had a high mortality rate.

Time went by, and the miraculous effects that had been expected from the ingestion of yogurt were late in coming; the suspected longevity of Bulgarian peasants turned out to be a naive myth. Shortly after, the theory of colic intoxication, following countless other theories, went out of fashion and ceased to interest the medical establishment.

Voronoff's Gorilla Testicles

The more illustrious and important the patients were, the more the impossible was attempted to keep them alive: The Duke of Guise, dismayed by the useless cures that were forced on Francis II, took his physicians to task, astounded "that medicine could not do more for the life of a king than for [that of] an old peasant."

History repeats itself: In the 1950s, a famous Swiss clinician whose methods smacked of quackery gave Pius XII injections of a rare and costly serum made from the live cells of a lamb's fetus, in the hopes of curing the pope's tumor of the stomach; the press carried the sensational announcement that the pope had recovered, but it turned out that the tumor had never existed.

As the science of medicine advanced by strides, it started a race to prolong life at any cost, a rational denial of decadence and a biological end. The newest scientific magic turned to the endocrine system, the regulator and balancer of bodily functions. At the end of the nineteenth century, it was discovered that many small glands such as the hypophysis, formerly believed to be of little use, secrete potent substances called hormones; some of these, present in the sexual glands, seemed able to dominate the process of aging even when present in tiny amounts. Therefore, all that was necessary was to refurnish the body with these hormones. In 1899, Brown Séquard, an elderly French physiologist, injected himself with extract of dog's testicles. Though the injections caused painful abscesses in his buttocks, he claimed that he had received an immediate rejuvenation and even had himself photographed after the experiments, yet any modest charlatan could have told him that his reacquired youth was only a figment of suggestion.

His theories were taken up again by Serge Voronoff, a scientist so esteemed that he had been nominated director of the experimental laboratory of the College of France. Borrowing ideas from the naturalist Buffon, who had observed cases of exceptional longevity in animals, Voronoff was sure that a man could live to the age of 140.[10] During his sojourn in Egypt he had noticed that some eunuchs, castrated while still very young, had aged precociously: Their breasts drooped like those of old grandmothers, and their spirits and energies were diminished. This was enough for him to formulate: "The testicles are the only distributors of energy that stimulate the immense beehive of sixty trillion cells that make up our bodies; only when the sexual glands retain a sufficient number of active cells is the physical decline of man retarded; only the grafting of sexual glands can restore the vigor and clearness of mind of youth, because each person is as good as the condition of his testicles." "On a des couilles ou on n'en a pas!" ("Either one has balls or one does not") was a motto in fashion amongst the French military.[9]

In Italy as elsewhere, Voronoff's cure had immediate success, and his followers began injecting patients with chimpanzee and gorilla testicles. This treatment was satisfying to many, because it supported the theory that the secret of longevity lay only in male sexual hormones and had nothing to do with moderate conduct. Voronoff insisted that a person with many vices could live a long time as long as he had a sufficient production of hormones.[10]

After a while, it was obvious that the histrionic old doctor had confused his desires with reality, and soon his patients became once again, as the Sicilians say, "old moths." Voronoff was right only when he blamed his failures on the incredulous and pessimistic attitude of his patients. If he had glanced at one of the chapters in Leonardo Fioravanti's *Fisica* he would have read: "[T]hose who have practiced coitus too much are made to eat Rooster's balls..." but, the great charlatan warns, "the substance of the Rooster lies in the blood ... and this restores nature more than if ten Roosters with their balls be eaten in a week!"[12]

Nicola Pende, the father of modern endocrinology, remembered a charlatan who called himself the "Wizard of Cerignola." This man had a dazzling intuition: nothing would attract young southern Italian men about to get married more than a cure that would increase their sexual drive. This neo–Voronoff, after giving the aspiring bridegrooms a short lesson on sexology, proposed expensive injections that supposedly contained an extract of a young bull's testicles. With professional superciliousness, he prepared before their eyes a large syringe with which he aspirated a yellowish liquid. Once the patient was lying face down, he rapidly exchanged the full syringe for an empty one and gave a deep injection with its long needle. He was so confident of the real success of his treatment that when at last he was discovered and denounced, he confused the judges by calling numerous young men who testified that after the treatment, they had obtained an admirable boost in their sexual performances.

One of the last alchemists of our century, the Rumanian doctor Ana Aslan, introduced a medicine, "Gerovital H-3," which she claimed would stop the wear of time and revitalize the whole body. This modern electuary's fame spread through most of the Western world with undeniable success; in countries where it was not authorized for sale, it was bought by eager clients on the black market. Elegant clinics opened where rejuvenation was promised: Many successful physicians and scientists declared that they had tested the properties of the drug — a simple vasodilative with a base of procaine — not only on their patients, but on themselves, with incontrovertible success. Suggestion and clever advertising convinced patients, and the doctors who tried it, of its marvelous effects. After a time,

Gerovital H-3, like the celebrated Erbolate, was quickly forgotten, but other remedies lie waiting to enchant minds and breed new hopes.

Now it seems that the relentless passage of the years can be checked with some of the latest discoveries that lie on the shelves in pharmacies: megavitamins, minerals, antioxidants, often wrapped in enticing packets, usually prescribed in massive doses. Today the patient's choice is still manipulated by cunning salespeople who preach insolent errors, make false promises, and distort reality, encouraged by an enormous pharmaceutical market in continuous expansion. The philosopher of science, Popper, wrote in our day: "But in politics as in medicine, those who promise too much are almost always quacks."

Theories pass quickly, and therapeutic deceptions are not often discovered promptly. The ultimate hope for the third millennium is resurrection, no longer mystical, but biological. If the fault of aging is not our own, but a destiny written in our genes, we can be reborn, perhaps choosing more pleasing physical characteristics: the color of our hair and eyes, our height. In this manner, we have been robbed of serenity and the acceptance of death. And yet we should keep in mind the legend of Eos, the golden-haired, rosy-fingered goddess of dawn, and her mortal lover Tithonos. She pleaded with Zeus to grant him immortality but forgot to ask that he be given eternal youth in the bargain. And Zeus, since he was a jealous god, gave Tithonos immortality, but he included old age, a fate more terrible even than death. As his hair began to turn gray and his limbs began to lose their vigor, Eos became ashamed of his company; for a time she let him roam her palace and feed on ambrosia, but finally, when he was reduced to only a feeble voice, she locked him in his chamber, where he can still be heard, babbling endlessly on.

The words of the Japanese poet Kenko Yoshida, written in the early fourteenth century, are worth remembering: "[T]he beauty of life is in its impermanence ... yet for such as love the world, a thousand years would fade like the dream of one night."

CHAPTER 14

"It is said that Medicine is of two parts: one is called a physician's science, the other is called Art"*

Orthodox or Alternative Medicine: A False Problem

Concerned with defending their prestige and the benefits of their profession, physicians have tried to find a rational explanation for the success of quackery, the dark shadow that has always accompanied the practice of medicine along its long and difficult path.

Scipione Mercuri had no doubts: Only the devil could have invented the "infamous art" of quackery. The Great Tempter, who proffered "lies and apples" to our forefathers in the Garden of Eden, is the ancestor of quacks; these follow his example, mount their platforms, tell tall stories, and deceive the populace, selling "rubbish and other things." The same master of deceit who prodded man toward a life of vice and sin now goads charlatans to their constant wandering, to their depraved habits: "with zanys, with puppets, ... with prostitutes, some to the sound of a lyre, some to a lute, or a harp."[2]

Universal opinion, still shared in our own times, holds that it is not

---

*"La medisina si ditta in due cosse: uno modo si ditta instrumento de medego, lo altro modo si ditta Arte."— From the introduction to a fourteenth-century codex containing Rolando di Parma's *Cyrugia*.[1]

217

the devil, but rather ignorance that shoves people into the arms of quacks: A fantastic hypothesis, a miraculous remedy, an absurd promise to provide eternal health, youth, and beauty is immediately believed by a credulous and naive public.

In 1500, Cosimo Aldana, nicknamed "The Spaniard," for his origin, wrote a dissertation brimming with resentment and full of insults against "The Wicked Vulgar Herd"; he maintained that the real cause of quackery lay in the lack of manners and education of the populace: a riffraff made up of "slow and stupid minds," who prefer to listen to "those second-rate doctors, or quacks, who succumb to the most vulgar daydreams instead of turning for advice to those who are very erudite."[3] The Spaniard pretended not to notice that even in his day the underprivileged and ignorant were not the only ones who bestowed success on quacks. Charlatans who could use words more skillfully than the sword had no difficulty in persuading high-ranking personalities, princes, nobles and even men of learning to take their fanciful baits.

It is easy to understand why people put their faith so willingly in charlatans during the centuries that were dominated by the medicine of humors, a time when doctors subjected their poor patients to interminable purges and vomiting, torrential enemas, cauterizations and pitiless bloodlettings, and imperiously ordered useless remedies for diseases that they did not even recognize. Yet even in our own times, transplants and biotechnologies notwithstanding, an instinctive clinging to much that is supernatural, a fascination for any new and different cure believed to be powerful and miraculous, are traits so deeply rooted in human nature that they still favor every form of quackery.

From time immemorial, the desire to "practice medicine," the urge to heal, the readiness to proffer advice which can help our neighbors, or at least show our interest in their welfare, is a formidable incentive for the expansion of quackery. To offer medical advice is gratifying and satisfactory, often an attempt to emerge or an eagerness to earn the gratitude and respect of others.

Gonnella, the quick-witted jester with "a shiny round nose," whose sharp witticisms and profound wisdom were recounted by Matteo Bandello, made a bet with his lord, Nicolò III d'Este, Duke of Ferrara: He would demonstrate that medicine is the most practiced trade in the whole world. One morning early, the jester left home, his hat pulled down over his forehead, a large bandage around his cheek, a look of suffering on his face. The first person that he met asked him what had happened, and when Gonnella answered that he had a terrible toothache the man immediately offered his advice. The same scene repeated itself with every person he met along the way. When he arrived at the palace, he was surrounded by a crowd of guards and courtesans, who, in turn, advised every sort of remedy; even the duke ordered his court physician to prepare a special medicine, the most infallible of all. At that point, Gonnella, having easily won the wager, tore off his bandages.[4]

"Theologians die of hunger, physicists languish, astronomers are ridiculed, dialecticians are ignored: There is only the physician who gains more fortune than all the rest together," commented Erasmus of Rotterdam. "The principal advantage of medicine is this: The more he who practices it is ignorant, daring and reckless, the more he is esteemed by princes and lords."[5] And Roger Bacon observed, "In this art, ill faith triumphs, and the charlatan prevails over the wise. The power of vulgar opinion is such in the generality of mankind that often the charlatan is put before the illuminated and erudite physician. For this reason, the Ancients gave, as sister to Aesculapius, the sorceress Circe."[6]

"From the prince down to the basest man," noted Carlo Gandini, in his defiant criticism of Professor Tissot's book, "there is not a man who does not presume to have notions of Medicine, and that his own ideas are greatly superior to those of another." And he adds that many times he was forced to listen to people who talked of medicine, "prating without sense but obtaining the approval and consent of those present."[7]

The Importance of Suggestion

> Medicina illa benedicta
> Quae suo nomine solo…
> Surprenanti miraculo,
> Depuis si longo tempore
> Facit à gogo vivere
> Tant de gens omni genere…[8]
>
> (Blessed medicine
> Whose name alone…
> is a wondrous miracle.
> For so long a time
> it has let people of all kinds
> live in prosperity.)

Thus sang the Troupe du Roy, a ballet of eight attendants carrying syringes, six apothecaries, twenty-two doctors, and eight dancing surgeons, as they entered the stage on the evening of February 10, 1673, for the first representation of "Le Malade Imaginaire." Later, as the curtain went down, Jean Baptiste Poquelin, known as Molière, the man who with these desecrating verses had intended to unmask the deceptive fortunes of medicine, died, shaken by convulsions.

There is no doubt that medicine has provided, and still provides, unexpected opportunities for profit at the expense of the patient; this is the main reason, if not the only one, that has always attracted quacks. But the medical profession, if made the most of, can offer many other enticing privileges. In the seventeenth century, Bonardo Frattegiano listed amongst "Le Miserie" of being a physician, "having to rise in the middle of the night to visit the infirm, to gaze on their filth, to listen to their laments, sighs, spasms, pains, sometimes horrors, silences, and melancholy." But the benefits far outweigh the drawbacks. What can be more exhilarating, Frattegiano asks, than "imperiously commanding the loftiest princes, receiving monies without number, and by the handful, promising health to the infirm, and everyone needing him, and holding in hand the lives of all, and touching the pulse, the head, and the body of the most graceful maidens, and the most regarded matrons of the world, does this not seem marvelous happiness?"[9]

In the years before the last world war, many young people discovered their medical vocation after reading Cronin's "The Citadel," Axel Munthe's "The Story of San Michele," and Andrea Maiocchi's "Life of a Surgeon." The medical profession was a humanitarian choice of lofty social value and consigned other professions to the backstage. The aspiring doctors, having chosen like modern crusaders to fight disease and infinite miseries, were certain of dedicating their lives to something important and genuinely useful for those who suffered. At the end of their studies, photographs with the names of the graduates from medical school were exhibited in a showcase in one of the busiest streets in the city, immediately examined by mothers who had daughters of a marriageable age. On commencement day, after the congratulations of their teachers, the neograduates received from their proud and moved parents a fountain pen or a watch, indispensable instruments for their new profession.

A life of sacrifice and renunciation then began for the young doctor — a continuous succession of triumphs and losses. Science had taught him to be responsible for the physical condition of his patient, but it was art that imposed upon him the task of curing with a spirit of loyal and faithful solidarity. The family doctor was created in this manner, a paternal and consoling figure who was present at his patient's bedside during the most critical moments of his existence, giving support throughout the anxieties and uncertainties of his illness.

As the years went by, as medicine and surgery collected one incredible success after another, transplanting, substituting organs, modifying the laws of nature as they pleased, the number of specialists who were scientifically up to date grew without restraint; at the same time, those doctors who still practiced with intimate and deep understanding dwindled accordingly. At the university, students learned a limited model, in which human beings were considered complex biochemical machines and diseases were organized into giant statistics performed on laboratory mice. For a modern and rational professional, competence alone, and not art, was considered the most important virtue; trust, comfort, dialogue with the patient were discarded, considered a boring waste of time, a debasement of professional authority.

Diagnoses provided by complex instruments, although they have undeniable advantages, have helped to put even more distance between patient and doctor. The physician no longer needs to touch, listen, talk, or even meet the worried glance of his patient, who is left alone, without any emotional or cognitive support during the uncertainties and anxieties of an illness that he rightly considers his own individual problem. Diminished in his mystic and hallowed role, the doctor is viewed as being on the same level as an electronics technician; the patient, when he turns for help in resolving his physical and spiritual problems, can hardly tell the difference between his doctor's face and the screen of a computer. In a short time, with the progressive erosion of the bond between doctor and patient, the prestige that physicians have always enjoyed has begun its decline. In this manner, a medical procedure becomes a simple business transaction, which does not require gratitude, which can be publicly challenged and even brought before the courts of law. Diffidence and hostility often separate doctors from their patients, and this infected atmosphere degenerates into bad sanitary practice, public denunciations and a complete lack of trust or reciprocal respect.

During the present era of medical miracles, we are spectators of a paradoxical phenomenon: a large part of the public takes shelter in so-called alternative medicines, a phenomenon that regards medicine alone and no other science. During this period of scientific medicine's highest splendor, an ever-expanding avalanche of healers, homeopaths, mesotherapists, dietitians, acupuncturists, mesmerists, pranotherapists, histrionic magicians, and religious and mystic faith healers find such favor with the public that they often support florid business activities.

When confronted at times by the undeniable achievements of these creators of false Utopias, there is no point in anxiously trying to prove that their accomplishments are falsehoods or illusions skillfully prepared by shrewd charlatans. It is fruitless to demonstrate that biological activity cannot exist in the endless dilutions prepared by a homeopathic doctor: It is the spiritual void left by the orthodox physician that he fulfills after a lengthy and pondered visit; he bases himself more on intuition than on real facts, attaching importance to subjective symptoms, and he obtains a positive effect by assuring an improvement, even if temporary, or a recovery, either apparent or real.

At the end of the last century, a British survey on unorthodox medical cures pointed out that charlatan healers spent eight times more time with their patients than did licensed physicians. A few years later, an international congress, held in Berlin for the study of the spreading scourge of quackery, reported that a third of these healers obtained results without using instruments or proposing remedies, but by "sympathy alone." An explanation for these strange results should be looked for in the progressive deconsecration of the medical act. Throughout these obscure practices, often smacking of quackery, the patient listens to words of assurance, unconsciously hoping to find the lost and reassuring figure of a family doctor, a personal healer to be exchanged for the hurried specialist imposed by collective medicine.

The contrast between alternative and orthodox medicine is actually a false problem, because medicine, understood as both an art and a science, can only be one: that which strives to cure the patient, or at least help him feel better. If "Health is the silence of the organs," as Leriche once maintained, any treatment that procures physical or moral well-being has the right to be considered a useful remedy. We cannot but agree with Isabelle Stengers, who recently said that a suffering body is not a reliable witness for the efficacy of a treatment, because it can heal even for the wrong reasons.[10]

Medicine's lengthy and difficult progress was not made of scientific discoveries and clinical triumphs alone: It is also a history of obscurantism, dogmatism, false ethics, and great greed. The lobotomies practiced on mental patients by the neurosurgeon Moniz in the twentieth century assuredly caused more damage than the pretend operations, superficial cuts on the forehead, performed by charlatans in the seventeenth century when they pretended to extract, with a rapid sleight of hand, a small stone, the "pierre de folie" from the head of a deranged person. This does not justify an attempt to condone quackery, because most of these likable adventurers used every kind of fraud to procure themselves facile gain, nor is it sufficient to insist that charlatans sold many useful substances taken from a wealth of herbal thaumaturgy. The most useful secret that we have inherited from charlatans is not the recipe for some potent remedy, but the demonstration of the incomparable power of suggestion: a word that in medicine has always conjured up an idea of dependency, influence, often fraudulent and malicious, artfully provoked by a bewitching individual on a person with a weak and confused mind.

Yet all the magical and religious sources of the art of medicine have their foundations in suggestion: Without its valid assistance it would be impossible to explain the fact that for many centuries the useless, fanciful remedies of the medicine of humors (theriaca, or the charlatans' false concoctions, such as orvietan), demonstrated their validity and their confirmed efficacy on countless generations of patients. On the other hand, how can we believe that all of our distant ancestors were foolish enough to continue, for over a thousand years, a remedy if it had constantly failed to produce the requested results? Even the lowliest merchant of remedies or the most grotesque scoundrel who performed on a platform, selling his stones, amulets, unguents, elixirs, juleps and plasters with histrionic gestures and bombastic rhetoric, contributed to the demonstration that an irrational choice and the absence of any scientific value in a medicine does not always correspond to a lack of efficacy.

In the twentieth century, other panaceas, other illusions, not dissimilar from those offered by charlatans, have produced beneficial effects: Millions of people believed that they could regain their health and strength by sipping tonics; trusting masses received daily intravenous injections of calcium chloride as protection against tubercular infection; many students, before facing exams, were certain that they could recuperate their intellectual faculties by taking phosphorus pills.

The idea that suggestion, considered a mysterious and obscure deceit, can avert or defeat an illness is very difficult to accept, as it is so far removed from science and rationality. "But suggestion," identifiable in the placebo effect, "takes no notice of logic or reason: it delights in irrationality in order to better deceive that which is called the unfathomable credulity of human beings."[11]

Now even scientists realize that a change is coming about. The latest spectacular research in neurophysiology is about to demonstrate that suggestion can act with a verified biological activity; it can become a significant element in helping or accelerating healing or in providing temporary relief, especially when scientific medicine can offer no real hope of cure. Just as sentiments, hidden passions, secret conflicts, negative events in life can be at the origin of many illnesses, so the protective function of many alternative cures is undeniable. A belief, a trusting hope, a desire for help which has been satisfied between healer and patient can provoke a positive emotional state and transform itself into a therapeutic agent which is sometimes so powerful that it can even determine modifications in the cells and tissues, induce mechanisms of immunity which are able to cause a sense of well-being: All these positive factors, as yet incompletely understood, can aid the process of healing.

In a near future, the physician will not have any autonomous function in formulating a diagnosis or deciding the therapy that needs to be undertaken. He will be able to regain the mystic qualities of a healer only if he is able to reestablish this ancient suggestive relationship with his patient, a relationship charged with compassion, feeling, and fruitful dialogue; if he will remain faithful to the teachings of Leonardo Fioravanti, the prince of charlatans, when he reminded doctors that "the most salutary medicine is in the word." Little or nothing has changed in the human mind. For this reason, the suggestion of Louis Patin, illustrious physician of the Medical Faculty of Paris in the seventeenth century, is still valid: He maintained the paradox that quackery should be included as a subject to be taught to medical students.

Autopsy of a Charlatan

"[I]n order to uncover the vagus or pneumogastric nerve in the lateral region of the neck, it is necessary to incise the skin, the superficial layer of the connective tissue, the superficial and deep fascia, until reaching the carotid sheath in which it is held, along with the common carotid artery and the internal jugular vein. Care must be taken when incising the resistant fibrous sheath...." On a gray autumn afternoon in 1942, a student repeated his notes out loud to his companion before facing the practical exam on a cadaver, observed by Professor Massart, the brilliant young head teaching assistant of the Institute of Human Anatomy in Pisa.

If the difficult dissection were a success, if the blessed nerve were uncovered without problems, it would be a big step toward surmounting the next, dreaded, oral examination. The two students cringed at the thought that in a few days they would find themselves standing before the professor of human anatomy, a small man whose long white hair framed a lean and nervous face adorned with a thin mustache which he fretfully twisted at each incorrect answer; renowned for his legendary severity, even his way of dressing recalled the famous anatomists of the nineteenth century: long black jacket, bow tie on a stiff, starched collar, striped pants beneath which appeared small black shoes half covered by spats. The young men were fully aware how difficult it would be to pass this exam: Over half

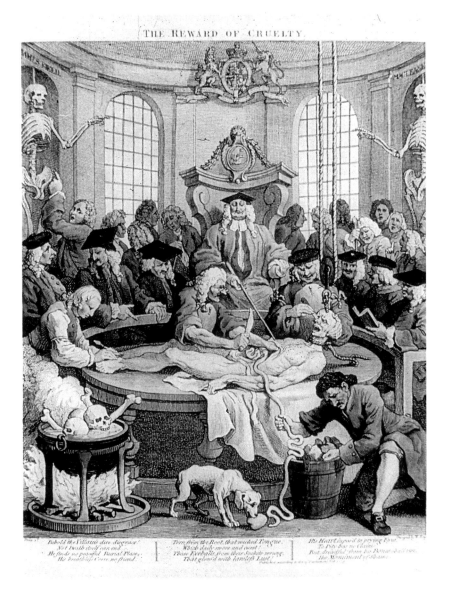

The Reward of Cruelty. Satire of an autopsy. Engraving by William Hogarth (1751). U.S. National Library of Medicine, Bethesda, MD.

of their fellow students had failed. There was a war, and those who were unable to finish the biennium exam would be faced with the nightmare of being drafted immediately.

When they had put on their white coats, retrieved their pincers, scalpels and probes from their black bags, they slipped their hands into rubber gloves, a rare commodity at the time; then they entered the dissecting room, stoically resigned to the subtle stench of rotting corpses and the acrid odor of formaldehyde that took away their breath.

On the marble tables lay two cadavers, both missing their legs, which had been used for other dissections; one of these rigid trunks, by now drained of blood, belonged to a young woman, the other to a wiry old man. Each one had a long incision on the abdomen, hastily sewn with string, a sign that their internal organs had been removed. The two candidates chose the old man, because his extreme leanness would facilitate the dissection. First, they laterally extended as far as possible the rigid neck of the body, which even in its corrupted matter seemed to retain a certain dignity, almost as if it were detached from its own death. Careful to avoid dangerous cuts, they began to slit the tissues, and the dissection proceeded, slowly at first, but without particular difficulty.

Suddenly the lights went out, and the shriek of the anti–air-raid siren made the window panes rattle. Now the darkened room, barely lit by the stump of a candle, prevented the students from carrying on the dissection; it was a chance to relax and exchange a few words with the anatomy room attendant, a burly man with a strangely sweet voice which belied his trade of dismemberer of corpses. As the hours went slowly by, he told the students what he knew about the obscure lives of the wretched remains: Those of the female belonged to a young woman who had died of tuberculosis in the city's sanatorium; those of the old man had been brought, along with other corpses, from the insane asylum in Volterra. "He was," the attendant chuckled, "an old charlatan, a healer, who with his strange cures and remedies had been quite successful, before he was locked up as crazy." Then the attendant jokingly warned the two students to be very careful, since they were dissecting a colleague.

"Gentlemen, instead of laughing, you should take care," intervened Professor Massart, "for you will always have something to learn from a charlatan in your clinical practice, in your relationship with future patients; while you are practicing on corpses, he would have been able to teach you something about the art of healing. In any case, you owe him respect, for in his own way, alive or dead, he attempted to decipher the many unsolved enigmas that concern healing and disease."

The lights went back on; the vagus nerve, a thin gray thread, was finally uncovered and laid out on the probe. Again the room was silent; the two students imagined that they saw a thin smile on the livid lips of the old man, as his half-closed eyes stared at them, brimming with mystery.

Glossary of Herbs
and Medical Ingredients

Absinthe: the oil of the wormwood, of Persian origin. Used as a stomachic and tonic.

Aconite, or wolf's bane, also called napellus: a highly poisonous plant that grows in wild rocky places; used against fever and neuralgia.

Alum: a double sulfate formed by the union of potassium sulphate and crude aluminum sulphate. Soluble in water, it is a powerful astringent, used for toothache, and to strengthen the gums, or as a hemostatic; often applied to severed blood vessels.

Amber: "the ancients gave it the name of succinum, from succus, juice. Often imagined as a concretion of the tears of birds, or urine of a beast. Amber assumes all figures in the ground; that of a pear, an almond, a pea; and among others there have been found letters very well formed, and even Hebrew and Arabick characters. White amber is used for medicinal purposes."

Angelica: a plant native of rivers and wet ditches in northern Europe; also cultivated for its strong and agreeable aromatic odor. The name derives from its supposed magical virtues.

Anise: a plant originally indigenous to Egypt. When distilled in water, it yields a volatile, syrupy, fragrant oil.

Antimony: "a mineral substance of a metalline nature. Basil Valentine, a German monk, gave some to his fellow monks as a purge, and they all died, hence the name antimoine (antimonk)."

Aqua fortis: "a corrosive liquor made by distilling purified nitre with calcined vitriol, or rectified oil of vitriol in a strong heat. The liquor, which rises in fumes, is red as blood. It dissolves all metals except gold, but if sea salt is added, it becomes aqua regia and dissolves no metal but gold."

Asphodel: a plant of the lily kind. The particular plant of the dead, its pale blue blossoms are believed to cover the meadows of Hades.

Baccaris: a plant whose aromatic root yields an oil occasionally used as a remedy in diseases of the lungs and as a demulcent.

Balsam or **Balm of Peru:** the product of a leguminous tree from San Salvador. In medicine it is a stimulating ointment and relieves asthma and coughs.

Camphor: a whitish, translucent, volatile substance with a peculiarly penetrating odor and an aromatic cooling taste. Common or laurel camphor is distilled from the wood of a lauracious tree, cinnamonum camphor, obtained from Formosa and Japan. It is of frequent use in medicine as a nervous stimulant and antispasmodic in typhoid and hysterical states.

Celandine, or **swallowwort,** also **"vincetoxicum":** a papaveraceous plant of Europe employed as a purgative and a remedy for warts. Its name derives from herba chelidonia, "having to do with swallows," because it was believed that swallows cured themselves with this plant.

Centaurea: a thistlelike plant similar to gentian, feigned to have cured a wound on the foot of the centaur Chiron. The root was used as a eupeptic depurant. Centaurea benedicta was highly valued as a counterpoison.

Cinchona: so called after the Countess of Cinchon, vice-queen of Peru, who in 1638 was cured of a fever by using cinchona bark. The bark of this evergreen tree is valuable as a remedy for fever and a tonic; quinine is an alkaloid which is obtained from the bark.

Diacatholicum: a purge for all humors, composed of many ingredients.

Diafinicum: a purge made of date pulp.

Diaprunis: a lenitive or solutive electuary made from powdered prunes.

Elderberry: the purplish-black fruit of the elder, sambucus nigra, used for making a kind of wine, used as an aperient and a diuretic.

Dragon's blood: a red resinous juice of an East Indian tree, the calamus draco, used as an astringent.

Fraxinella, or **dittany:** a plant that grows on Mount Dicte in Crete. Its oil is so volatile that the air around it is said to become inflammable on hot summer days. "The Hart, perced with the Dart, runneth out of hand to the hearb Dicatanum and is healed."

Galbanum: gum resin in the form of translucent tears, obtained from a species of ferula in the desert regions of Persia; used as a stimulating expectorant and an ingredient in plasters.

Galega, or **goat's rue:** tall, leguminous herbs with blue or white flowers. Used as a diaphoretic and stimulant.

Gentian: named after the Illyrian king Gentius, who discovered its properties. The root, extremely bitter and without astringency or acridity, is used in pharmacology and as a tonic.

Gratiola: low herbs with small flowers, named from the Latin "gratia" for its medicinal virtues. It has a bitter, acrid taste and is employed as a drastic purgative.

Guaiac: a greenish-brown resin obtained from the wood of the guaicum, a South American tree. Reputed as a diaphoretic and alterative, it was often prescribed in cases of gout and rheumatism.

Hyacinth: in ancient times, a gem of bluish-violet color, supposed to be the sapphire. Occasionally the word is used to indicate an electuary made of gems.

Imperatorin: a resin derived from the plant ostruthium, or master wort, which grows in wet pastures in Scotland.

Jasper: a bright-colored, translucent gem varying in color, but with green the most common. A highly esteemed precious stone, used in jeweled electuaries.

Juniper: the berries of this evergreen tree yield a volatile oil, used as a diuretic and stimulant.

Kaolin: a fine variety of clay, named for a hill in China on which it was found. It is pure white and one of the two ingredients in Oriental porcelain.

Mallow: a plant with soft, downy leaves and emollient properties.

Mercury: a metal which has the peculiar quality of remaining fluid at ordinary temperatures. Mercuric sublimate is a violent poison, used in medicine and extensively in surgery as an antiseptic, especially as a preservative for dressings of the skin.

Mullein: a tall weed, verbascum thapsus. An infusion is used in domestic practice for catarrh and dysentery.

Mummy: "the dried flesh of human bodies embalmed with myrrh and spice, or a liquor running from such mummies. Mummy has been esteemed resolvent and balsamick; besides it, the skull, and even the moss growing on the skulls, have been celebrated for antiepileptick virtues; the fat also of the human bodies has been recommended in rheumatisms."

Musk: an odoriferous substance secreted by the male musk deer, the strongest and most lasting of perfumes, it is also used in medicine as a diffusible stimulant and antispasmodic. Imported from Asia in the natural pods, or bags, it was frequently mixed with blood, fat and hairs.

Myrobalan, or **cherry plum:** the dried fruit of an Indian tree of the species Terminalia, greatly esteemed as a cure for diarrhea.

Myrrh: the balsamic juice of the Arabian myrtle. Used as an astringent tonic.

Nettle: a small plant with stinging hairs, used as a diuretic and astringent.

Nightshade, or **belladonna:** a poisonous plant which yields the alkaloid atropin. The plant and its alkaloid are largely used in medicine to relieve pain, to check spasm and excessive perspiration, and especially in surgery to dilate the pupil and paralyze the accommodation of the eye.

Olibanum, or **frankincense:** incense made from the gum resin of the tree Boswellia of Somalia.

Opium: "[T]he ancients were greatly divided about the virtue of opium, some calling it a poison and others the greatest of all medicines. At present it is in high esteem, and externally applied it is emollient, relaxing and discutient, and greatly promotes suppuration. Its first effect is the making of the patient cheerful, as if he had drunk moderately of wine; it removes melancholy, excites boldness, and dissipates the dread of danger; it afterwards quiets the spirits, eases pain, and disposes to sleep."

Opobalsam: a fragrant, resinous juice of the shrub commiphora opobalsamum. It was believed that it would grow only in Egypt and was so precious that it had to be defended day and night by armed guards. The same shrub produces myrrh.

Opoponax: a gum resin obtained from the roots of the plant opoponax chironium, used as an antispasmodic.

Pimpinella: a species of plant that produces anise or cumin.

Pinole: an aromatic powder used in Italy for making chocolate.

Plantain: a familiar yard weed with large spreading leaves. It has a soothing effect when bound on inflamed surfaces.

Plumbago or **leadwort:** often called **toothwort** for the use to which its caustic leaves or roots are put. It was sometimes used to produce blisters.

Potentilla: a small plant, similar to the wild strawberry, so called in allusion to its repute as a powerful medicine. The section of the genus known as tormentilla (from "torment") is highly astringent and was considered a remedy for toothache and a protection against plague.

Radish: used as an antiscorbutic.

Rhubarb: Originally native to Western China and Eastern Tibet, it reached Europe through Russia and Turkey and was named accordingly. It combines a cathartic with an astringent effect and is also used as a tonic and stomachic.

Rue: a plant with a strong, disagreeable odor, believed to ward off contagion. Stimulant and antispasmodic.

Sagapenum: a species of ferula from Persia. Yields a fetid gum resin, used for amenorrhea, hysteria.

Sandal: an aromatic resin, used as an incense.

Sandarac: a coniferous tree, callitris articulata, native of Morocco. Its transparent white resin, which forms in tears, was used as incense and was renowned for its medicinal properties.

Scabious, or **scabiosa:** a hairy, perennial herb which cures scaly eruptions. "Is not the rhubarb found where the sun most corrupts the liver, and the scabious by the shore of the sea, that God might cure as soon as he wounds?" (Jeremy Taylor)

Scammony: the resin of a plant of the same name which grows in Syria and Asia Minor. It appears in commerce in greenish-gray or black cakes. An energetic cathartic, it has an acrid taste and smells like cheese.

Scilla: a lilylike plant also known as wild hyacinth. Its bulb was used as an expectorant and diuretic.

Spoonwort, or **scurvy grass:** an antiscorbutic, similar to cress.

Storax: the resin of this small tree has a fragrance similar to vanilla. Used as an expectorant and stimulant.

Terebinth: the resin from the terebinth tree. The oil is called turpentine.

Yarrow, or milfoil, "a thousand leaves": a grayish-green plant a foot or so high, used as a mild astringent and tonic.

Zedoary: an East Indian drug, the product of Curcuma Zedoaria. It is aromatic, with a strong camphoraceous flavor and the odor of ginger. In medicine it is used like ginger.

The definitions in quotation marks are taken from *Johnson's Dictionary: A Modern Selection*, edited by E. L. McAdam and George Milne (London: Cassel-Wellington House).

Source Notes

Chapter 1

1. Marc'Antonio Savelli, *Pratica Universale del Dottor Marc'Antonio Savelli da Modigliana: Opera altissima e necessaria ad ogni qualità di persona* (Florence: G. Cocchini, Stamperia della Stella, 1665), p. 411.

2. Scipione Mercuri (Mercurij), *Degli errori popolari d'Italia* (Padua: F. Bolzetta, 1645), book IV, p. 264.

3. Sebastiano Rossi, *La Sferza, satire piacevoli alla venetiana* (Venice: Pietro Zaniboni, 1604), p. 93.

4. Piero Camporesi, *Il Libro dei Vagabondi* (Turin: Nuova Universale Einaudi, 1973), pp. 50–51.

5. *Ibid.*, p. 114.

6. State Archives of Naples, *Pragmaticae, Edicta, Decreta*, Titolus XCV (Naples: Officina Typographica Jacopi Raillad, 1682), p. 722.

7. Fynes Moryson, *An Itinerary*, quoted in C.M. Cipolla, *Cristofano e la Peste* (Bologna: Il Mulino, 1976), p. 295.

8. Tomaso Garzoni da Bagnocavallo, *La Piazza Universale di tutte le Professioni del Mondo* (Venice: Vincenzo Sonnesca, 1595), p. 757.

9. Benedetto Croce, *I Teatri di Napoli* (Bari: G. Laterza, 1966), pp. 107–108.

10. Mercuri, *Degli errori popolari d'Italia*, op. cit., p. 266.

11. Giuseppe Pitrè, *Medici, Chirurghi: Speziali Antichi in Sicilia* (Casa Editrice del Libro Italiano, 1941), p. 175ff.

12. Alberto Garosi, *Medici, Speziali, Cerusici e Medicastri nei Libri del Protomedicato Senese* (Siena: "Bollettino Senese di Storia Patria," Lazzeri, 1935), pp. 3–14.

13. Piero Camporesi, "Speziali e Ciarlatani" in *Cultura Popolare dell'Emilia Romagna* (Milan: Cassa di Risparmio e delle Banche del Monte Sivano, ed., 1981), p. 146ff.

14. Franco Cardini, quoted by Aldo Santini in "Società e Cultura" (Leghorn: *Il Tirreno*, Dec. 17, 1999), p. 12.

15. State Archives of Siena, Studio, f. 89, 1789.

16. Mauro Randone, "Studio Storico sui medici ciarlatani" (in *Minerva Medica* [varia] 55, 1964), pp. 589–602.

17. Nicola Latronico, *Un ciarlatano del '700 e i suoi contrasti col Magistero della Sanità* (Castalia, no. 7, 1946), pp. 445–459.

18. State Archives of Florence, Ufficiali di Sanità, f. 139, May 12, 1630.

19. Pitré, *Medici, Chirurghi, Speziali*, op. cit., p. 117.

20. Savelli, *Pratica Universale*, op. cit., p. 248.
21. Garzoni, *La Piazza Universale*, op. cit., p. 757.
22. *Gazzetta Toscana*, 1780, no. 7, p. 89.
23. State Archives of Venice, *Supplica al Serenissimo Principe del ProtomedicatoVeneto*, May 20, 1695, no. 2, p. 132.
24. State Archives of Venice, 1604, p. 129.
25. *Ibid.*, p. 133.
26. Anton Maria Cospi, *Il Giudice Criminalista* (Venice: Menafoglio, 1681), p. 372.
27. Garosi, *Medici, Speziali, Cerusici e Medicastri*, op. cit., p. 1.
28. State Archives of Siena, Studio, f. 58, 1672.
29. "Nuovo Bando a previsione in materia di Peste da osservarsi nella città e nella Contà di Bologna. Pubblicato in Bologna il 13 Novembre, 1629, Reiterato alli 14 del medesimo," Italian Broadsides concerning Public Health (New York: Mount Kisco, 1986. p. x.
30. State Archives of Florence, Ufficiali di Sanità, f. 150, August 1630, p. 219.

Chapter 2

1. *Gazzetta Toscana*, 1778, no. 51, p. 173.
2. Thomas Coryat, *Crudities, Travels in France and Italy* (Glasgow: James MacLehose and Sons, 1905), vol. I, pp. 409–412.
3. Ben Jonson, *Volpone*, Act II, Sc. II (New Haven, Conn.: Yale Univ. Press).
4. Giuseppe Giacchino Belli, *Il Ciarlatano* (Milan: L. Ferriani, 2nd ed., 1960), p. 31.
5. Ptolemy Tompkins, *The Monkey in Art* (New York: M. T. Train, Scala Books, 1994), p. 33.
6. *Il Mercato delle Maraviglie della Natura ovvero Istoria Naturale del Cavalier Nicolò Serpetro* (Venice: Tomasini, 1653), p. 292.
7. Croce, *I Teatri di Napoli*, see Chap. 1, note 9, p. 104.
8. Garzoni, *La Piazza Universale*, see Chap. 1, note 8, pp. 757–758.
9. Andrea Corsini, *Medici Ciarlatani e Ciarlatani Medici* (Bologna: Zanichelli, 1922), p. 417.
10. State Archives of Florence, Otto di Guardia e Balia del Principato, 1627, f. 2359.
11. Giovan Domenico Ottonelli, *Della Christiana Moderazione del Theatro Libro detto l'Ammonizioni s' Recitanti Per avvisare ogni Christiao à moderarsi da gli eccessi del recitare* (Florence: Giov. Antonio Bonardi, Alle Scale di Badia, 1652), p. 455ff.
12. Ibid., p. 417.
13. Croce, *I Teatri di Napoli*, see Chap. 1, note 9, p. 107.
14. Ottonelli, *Della Christiana Moderazione del Theatro*, op. cit., p. 440.
15. Piero Camporesi, *La Miniera del Mondo* (Milan: A. Mondadori, 1990), p. 143.
16. Ottonelli, *Della Christiana Moderazione del Theatro*, op. cit., p. 424.
17. Mercuri, *Degli Errori Popolari d'Italia*, see Chap. 1, note 2, p. 234.
18. Ottonelli, *Della Christiana Moderazione del Theatro*, op. cit., p. 425.
19. Mercuri, *Degli Errori Popolari d'Italia*, see Chap. 1, note 2, p. 234.
20. Pier Andrea Mattioli, *I Discorsi ... né sei libri di Pedacio Dioscoride Anarzabeo della Materia Medicinale* (Venice: Pezzana, ed., 1744), vol. VI, p. 205.
21. Coryat, *Crudities*, op. cit., p. 294.
22. Moryson, *An Itinerary*, see Chap. 1, note 7, p 425.
23. Corsini, *Medici Ciarlatani e Ciarlatani Medici*, op. cit., pp. 102–103.
24. Nicola Latronico, *Il ciarlatanesimo medico al tribunale di Sanità dello Stato di Milano* (Milan: "L'Ospedale Maggiore"), Sept., 1941, p. 391.
25. Thomas Sonnet De Courval, *Satyre contre les Charlatans et pseudomédicins empiriques* (Paris: Jean Millot, 1610), p. 59.
26. Piero Camporesi, *Il Paese della Fame* (Bologna: Il Mulino, 1978), p. 231.

Chapter 3

1. *Parere del Signor Lionardo di Capua divisato in otto Ragionamenti* (Naples: Antonio Bulison, 1681), p. 477.

2. Garzoni, *La Piazza Universale*, see Chap. 1, note 8, p. 743.

3. Anton Francesco Bertini, *La Medicina difesa dalle Calunnie degli Uomini Volgari e dalle Opposizioni de'Dotti* (Lucca: Marescandoli, 1699), pp. 119–120.

4. State Archives of Florence, Presidenza del Buon Governo, Affari Comuni, *Processo contro Lorenzo Bianchini*, 1784, no. 3.

5. Don Alessio Piemontese (pseudonym of Girolamo Ruscelli), *De' Secreti* (Venice: Alessandro Gardena, 1580), p. 123.

6. Ioannes Colle Bellunensis, *De Fascinatione in pueris, et in adultis in genere et in Specie, in Methodus Facile Parandi Iucunda, Tuta & Nova Medicamenta* (Venice: Apud Evangelistam Deuchinum, 1628), p. 191ff.

7. Mauro Randone and Pierluigi Ponti, "Un metodo di cura del '700: Le pillole di mercurio di Agostino Belloste," (*Minerva Medica*, 1966), p. 267ff.

8. State Archives of Florence, Presidenza del Buon Governo, Affari Comuni, 1784, no. 5.

9. Garzoni, *La Piazza Universale*, see Chap. 1, note 8, p. 114–116.

10. State Archives of Siena, Processi (Trials), 1748, f.za 59, p. 29ff.

11. Garzoni, *La Piazza Universale*, see Chap. 1, note 8, p. 843.

12. *Ibid.*, p. 825.

13. Leonardo Fioravanti, *La Cirurgia* (Venice: Heirs of Melchiorre Sessa, 1570), p. 127.

14. Lorenzo Gualino, *Storia Medica dei Romani Pontefici* (Turin: Minerva Medica, ed., 1934), p. 401.

15. *Gazzetta Toscana*, 1771, no. 30, p. 110.

Chapter 4

1. Alberico Benedicenti, *Malati, Medici, e Farmacisti* (Milan: U. Hoepli, 1924), vol. I, p. 499.

2. Don Silvio Boccone, *Museo di Fisica e di Esperienze, variato e decorato di Osservazioni naturali, Note medicinali, e Ragionamenti secondo i principi dé moderni* (Venice: Battista Zuccato, 1697), p. 111.

3. Charles McKay, *Memoirs of Extraordinary Popular Delusions* (London: R. Bentley, New Burlington Street, 1841. New edition published in 1980 by Harmony Books, New York), pp. 576–577.

4. Don Silvio Boccone, *Museo di Fisica e di Esperienze*, op. cit., p. 112.

5. Margaret Visser, *The Rituals of Dinner* (New York: Grove Weidenfeld, 1991), p. 56.

6. Leonardo Fioravanti, *Il Reggimento della Peste* (Venice: Heirs of Melchiorre Sessa, 1571), p. 231.

7. Girolamo Dian, *Cenni Storici sulla Farmacia Veneta* (Venice: Filippi, ed., 1900), pp.216–21.

8. Pietro Andrea Mattioli, *I Discorsi ... ne' sei libri di Pedacio Dioscoride Anarzabeo della Materia Medicinale* (Venice: Pezzan ed., 1744), vol. VI.

9. Francesco Redi, *Scritti di Botanica, Zoologia e Medicina*, edited by P. Polito (Milan: Longanesi e C., 1975), p. 67.

10. Garzoni, *La Piazza Universale*, see Chap. 1, note 8, p. 321.

11. Ottonelli, *Della Christiana Moderazione del Theatro*, see Chap. 2, note 11 (chapter III, Ammonitione IIIa, Warning no. III), p. 412.

12. Alessandro Tassoni, quoted in "Il Giardino d'Esculapio," October, 1935, p. 30.

13. Corsini, *Medici Ciarlatani e Ciarlatani Medici*, see Chap. 2, note 9, p. 44.

14. *Il Mercato delle Meraviglie*, see Chap. 2, note 6, p. 184.

15. Mattioli, *I Discorsi nei sei libri di Pedacio Dioscoride*, op. cit., p. 740.

16. Colle Bellunensis, *De Fascinatione in Pueris, et in adultis*, op. cit., pp. 183–210.

17. Don Silvio Boccone, op. cit., p. 93.

18. Francesco Redi, *Esperienze diverse intorno a cose naturali e particolarmente a quelle che si sono portate dalle Indie*, in F. Redi's notebooks on natural history, edited by O. Livi (Florence: Le Monnier, 1858), p. 175.

19. Serpetro, *Il Mercato delle Meraviglie*, op. cit., pp. 183–184.

20. Gio. Battista Fidelissimi da Pistoia, *Centurie d'Osservazioni Thaumaphysiche* (Bologna: Bartolomeo Cochi, 1619), pp. i–ii.

21. Serpetro, *Il Mercato delle Meraviglie*, see Chap. 2, note 6, p. 202.

22. Ulysses Aldrovandi, *Serpentum et Dracorum Hystoriae*, vol. II (Bononiae, apud Clementem Ferronium, 1630), pp. 373–374.

23. Achille Forti, *Il Basilisco ecc. Contributo alla Storia della Ciarlataneria*, Atti del Reale Istituto Veneto di Scienze, Lettere ed Arti (Acts of the Royal Venetian Institute for Science, Letters, and the Arts), Academic Year 1928-1929, vol. LXXXVIII; pp.229-233.

24. Mattioli, *I Discorsi ... né sei libri di Pedacio Dioscoride*, see Chap. 4, note 8, p. 801.

25. Serpetro, *Il Mercato delle Meraviglie*, see Chap. 2, note 6, p. 205.

26 . "Il Giardino d'Esculapio," 1959, no.1, p. 44.

27. Andrea M. Bacci, *Discorso sull'Alicorno* (Florence: Giorgio Marescotti, 1582), pp. 121–158.

Chapter 5

1. Celio Malespini, *Ducento Novelle*, Novella LXXXVII, "Prodezze medicinali di Jacopo Coppa" (Venice: Al Segno dell'Italia, 1609), p. 299ff.

2. *Ibid.*, p. 301.

3. *Ibid.*, p. 306.

4. *Ibid.*, p. 307.

5. Leonardo Di Capua, *Pareri del Signor Lionardo di Capua*, see Chap. 3, note 1, p. 576.

6. Garzoni, *La Piazza Universale* , see Chap. 1, note 8, p. 159.

7. Gabriele De Zerbis, *De cautelis medicorum*, Italian translation by Clodonovo Mancini in *Un codice deontologico del sec. XV* (Pisa: "Scientia Veterum," no. 44, 1913), p. 42.

8. Gianna Pomata, *La Promessa di Guarigione*, (Bari: Laterza e Figli, 1994), p. 87ff.

9. Adalberto Pazzini, *Medicina Denigrata* (Turin: Minerva Medica, 1948), p. 101.

10. Giovan Battista Morgagni, *Consulti medici*, edited by Enrico Benassi (Bologna: Cappelli, 1935), p. 178.

11. Ugo Viviani, *Vita, opere, iconografia e bibliografia di Francesco Redi* (Arezzo: Viviani, ed., 1924), p. 87.

12. Alberto Chiappelli, "I Primordi della Pubblicità Medica in Italia," (*Bollettino dell'Istituto Storico Italiano dell'Arte Sanitario*, no. 4, 1925), pp. 119–135.

13. Benedicenti, *Malati, Medici e Farmacisti*, see Chap. 4, note 1, p. 1006.

14. Bertini, *La Medicina difesa dalle Calunnie*, see Chap. 3, note 3, p. 100.

15. Ludovico Antonio Muratori, *Li tre Governi Politico, Medico, ed Ecclesiastico*, book II, *Il Governo Medico della Peste*, chap. I–III (Lucca: Domenico Ciuffetti e Filippo Maria Benedettini, 1743), p. 128ff.

16. *Ibid.*, p. 131.

17. Alberto Randone, "Studio Storico sui Medici Ciarlatani" (Turin: *Minerva Medica*, Various, 1953), p. 596.

18. *Avviso al Popolo intorno alla Sanità*, a work by Signor Tissot, translated from the French by Dr. Carlo Gandini (Milan: Federico Agnelli, 1770), chap. 35, pp. 189–210.

19. State Archives of Siena, Studio 59, Ciarlatani, *Foglietto d'Avviso al Pubblico del dottor Formigli detto l'Anonimo*, printed in Leghorn, 1752.

20. Johann Burkhard Mencken, *De Charlataneria Eruditorum*, edition of 1722. Republished in *The Charlatanry of the Learned* (New York: Alfred A. Knopf, 1937), p. iv, p. 164ff.

21. Gandini, *Avviso al Popolo intorno alla Sanità*, op. cit., notes on pp. 197 and 200.

Chapter 6

1. Leonardo Fioravanti, *Della Fisica*, (Venice: Stefano Curti, 1678), chap. XV, p. 158.

2. Leonardo Fioravanti, *La Cirurgia dell'Eccellente Dottore e Cavalier M. Leonardo Fioravanti Bolognese* (Venice: Heirs of Melchiorre Sessa, 1570), p. 178.

3. Leonardo Fioravanti, *Del Compendio de Secreti Universali* (Venice: Heirs of Melchiorre Sessa, 1572), p. 54.

4. *Dello Specchio di Scienza Universale dell'Ecc. Medico e Chirurgo M. Leonardo Fioravanti Bolognese* (Venice: Andrea Ravenoldo, 1567), p. 259.

5. Leonardo Fioravanti, *De'Capricci Medicinali* (Venice: Lodovico Avazo, 1565), p. 115.

6. Fioravanti, *Della Fisica*, op. cit., p. 163.

7. Leonardo Fioravanti, *Il Tesoro della Vita Umana* (Venice: Brigma, 1673), p. 310.

8. Fioravanti, *Della Fisica*, op. cit., pp. 338–339.

9. Fioravanti, *La Cirurgia*, op. cit., p. 320.

10. Fioravanti, *Del Compendio de' secreti universali*, op. cit., p. 54.

11. *Ibid.*, p. 150.

12. *Ibid.*, p. 147.

13. Fioravanti, *Il Tesoro della Vita Umana*, op. cit., p. 290.

14. Domenico Furfaro, *La vita e l'opera di Leonardo Fioravanti* (Bologna: Azzoguidi ed., 1963), p. 98.

15. Fioravanti, *Dello Specchio di Scienza Universale*, op. cit., p. 298.

16. Fioravanti, *Il Tesoro della Vita Umana*, op. cit., pp. 25–26.

17. *Ibid.*, p. 69.

18. Corsini, *Medici Ciarlatani e Ciarlatani Medici*, see Chap. 2, note 9, pp. 80–81.

19. Piero Camporesi, *La Miniera del Mondo* (Milan: "Il Saggiatore," A. Mondadori, 1990), p. 64.

20. Fioravanti, *Del Compendio de'secreti universali*, op. cit., p. 22.

21. Giuseppe A. Gentili , "Leonardo Fioravanti bolognese alla luce di ignorati documenti" (*Rivista delle Scienze Mediche e Naturali*, no. 1, January–June, 1951), pp. 16–41.

22. Salvatore De Renzi, *Storia della Medicina Italiana* (Naples, 1845; reprinted in Bologna by Forni, 1966), vol. III, p. 75.

23. Randone, *Studio storico su medici ciarlatani*, see Chap. 5, note 17, p. 596.

24. Davide Giordano, *Leonardo Fioravanti Bolognese* (Bologna-Trieste: L. Cappelli, ed., 1920), p. 20ff.

25. Giorgio Cosmacini, *Ciarlataneria e Medicina* (Milan: Raffaello Cortina, 1999), pp. 53–55.

Chapter 7

1. Belli, *Il Ciarlatano*, see Chap. 2, note 4, pp. 55–56.

2. John Camp, *Magic, Myth, and Medicine* (New York: Taplinger Publishing Co., 1974), p. 18.

3. Alberico Benedicenti, "Medicamenti rari e costosi dei tempi passati" (Milan: *Varietà Mediche*, Collezione Midy, ed. S.I.F.C.A, 2nd series, 1936), p. 10.

4. I. Wasserberger, *Contribution à l'Etude du Charlatanisme* (Paris: Bibliotèque Nationale), no. 8, T 4546, p. 621.

5. Gualino, *Storia Medica dei Romani Pontefici*, see Chap. 3, note 14, pp. 419–420.

6. *Ibid.*, p. 521.

7. *Parere del Signor Lionardo di Capua diviso in otto Ragionamenti*, op. cit., Ragion VII, (Reasoning no. VII), pp. 534–565.

8. Benedicenti, *Malati, Medici e Farmacisti*, see Chap. 4, note 1, p. 560.

9. Gualino, *Storia Medica dei Romani Pontefici*, see Chap. 3, note 14, p 60.

10. *Ibid.*, p. 62.

11. Piero Camporesi, *La Carne Impassibile* (Milan: "Il Saggiatore," 1983), p. 19.

12. Mattioli, *I Discorsi nei sei libri*, see Chap. 4, note 8, p. 564.

13. Cosmacini, *Ciarlataneria e Medicina*, see Chap. 6, note 25, p. 211.

14. "Quackery in the Past" (*The British Medical Journal*, May 27, 1911), pp. 1260–1261.

15. Corsini, *Medici Ciarlatani e Ciarlatani Medici*, see Chap. 2, note 9, p. 70.

16. Alberico Benedicenti, *Malati, Medici e Farmacisti*, see Chap. 4, note 1, p. 1006.

17. G. Doglia and F. Roagna, *I Secreti del Padre Auda* (Pisa: Gardini, ed., in *Scientia Veterum*, XVII, 1968), p. 152.

18. Fioravanti, *Il Tesoro della Vita Umana* , see Chap. 6, note 7, p. 51.

19. *Gazzetta Toscana delle Scienze Medico-Fisiche*, (no. 1, Feb. 15, 1843), pp. 167–172.

20. Dian, *Cenni Storici sulla Farmacia Veneta*, see Chap. 4, note 7, p. 50ff.

21. Benedicenti, *Malati, Medici e Farmacisti*, see Chap. 4, note 1, p. 1023.

22. Massimiliano Cardini, "Il Principe dei medicamenti del passato: La Triaca'"' (*Varietà Mediche*, no. 2, ed. S.I.F.C.A., Collezione Midy, Milan, 1934), pp. 2–14.

23. Dian, *Cenni Storici sulla Farmacia Veneta*, see Chap. 4, note 7, p.49ff.

24. *Ibid.*, p. 53.

25. *Ibid.*, p. 55.

26. Redi, *Esperienze diverse intorno a cose naturali e particolarmente a quelle che si sono portate dalle Indie*, see Chap. 4, note 9, p. 57.

27. *Secreti diversi e miracolosi racolti dal Falopia, e aprobati da altri medici di gran fama* (Venice: Alessandro Cardano, 1578), p. 104.

28. Boccone, *Museo di Fisica e di Esperienze*, see Chap. 4, note 2, p. 42.

29. Andrea Corsini, "Specifico e Ciarlatani d'altri tempi" (*Gazzetta Sanitaria* , no. 3, March, 1949), p. 108.

30. *Ibid.*, p. 109.

31. Leonardo Colapinto, "Segreti Farmaceutici e ciarlatani nei secoli XVII e XVIII" (*Atti e Memorie del Nobile Collegio Chimico-Farmaceutico di Roma*, 1965), p. 14.

32. Serpeto, *Il Mercato delle Meraviglie*, see Chap. 2, note 6, p. 43.

33. *Secreti Diversi e Miracolosi*, op. cit., Introduction, p. ii.

34. *Ibid.*, book III, p. 841.

35. *Maravigliosi Secreti di Medicina e Chirurgia dell'eccellente medico il Sig. Gio. Battista Zapata nuovamente ritrovati. Con l'aggiunta d'altri secreti raccolti dalli suoi Discepoli* (Rome: Tito, e Paolo Diani, 1536), p. 80.

36. *Secreti Diversi e Miracolosi*, op. cit., p. 120.

37. *Secreti Medicinali di M. Pietro Bairo di Torino, già medico di Carlo Secondo. Et questo libro, per l'utilità sua si chiama "Vieni Meco"* (Venice: Giacomo Cornetti, 1592), p. 124.

38. Don Alessio Piemontese, *Dé Secreti*, see Chap. 3, note 5, p. 42.

39. Garzoni, *La Piazza Universale*, see Chap. 1, note 8, p. 187.

Chapter 8

1. *La Fiera*, edited by P. Fanfani (Florence: Vallecchi ed.), vol. I, p. 519.

2. Francesco Vettori, "Viaggio in Alemagna" (1507), in *Historical Essays and Political Profiles*, edited by E. Niccolini (Bari: G. Laterza, 1972), pp. 31–32.

3. C. J. S. Thompson, *The Quacks of Old London* (London: Brentano, 1928), pp. 204–205.

4. Roy Porter, *Health for Sale: Quackery in England 1660–1850* (Manchester: Manchester University Press, 1989), chap. IV, p. 96.

5. Leslie G. Matthews, "Licensed Mountbanks in Britain" (*Pharm. Hist.*, 1972), no. II, p. 2.

6. Idem, "Italian Charlatans in England" (*Pharm. Hist.*, 1979), no. IX, chap. II, p. 7.

7. *Ibid.*, p. 3.

8. Porter, *Health for Sale*, op. cit., p. 99.

9. Matthews, *Licensed Mountbanks in Britain*, op. cit., pp. 38–39.

10. *Ibid.*, p. 40.

11. Mario Sensi, "Cerretani e ciarlatani nel secolo XV: Spigolature d'archivio" (*Medicina nei secoli*, 1978), no. 1, chap. III, pp. 282–284.

12. "Il Giardino d'Esculapio" (year XVI, no. 1, January, 1943), XXI, p. 24.

13. Luigi Rasi, *I Comici Italiani* (Florence: Fratelli Bocca, 1897), p. 555.

14. *Enciclopedia dello Spettacolo* (Rome: ed. Le Maschere), p. 169.

15. Croce, *I Teatri di Napoli*, see Chap. 1, note 9, pp. 104–105.

16. C. Sthéfen, Le Pamier, "L'Orvietan: histoire d'une famille des charlatans du Pont-Neuf aux XVII et XVIII siècle (Contugi)" (Paris: Lib. Illustréé, 1893).

17. Mario Battistini, "Medici ciarlatani e ciarlatani medici del sec. XVII. Il marchese Niccolò Cevoli Del Carretto in Francia e in Belgio" (*Rivista delle Scienze Mediche e Naturali*), nos. 7–8, July–August, 1936), XIV, pp. 243–255.

18. Giuseppe D'Amato, *Borri, uno Strawinski del Secolo XVII* (Rome: Casa del Libro, 1934), p. 21.

19. *Ibid.*, p. 69.

20. Giorgio Cosmacini, *Il Medico Ciarlatano: Vita Inimitabile di un Europeo del Seicento* (Rome-Bari: Laterza e Figli, 1998), pp. 66–67.

21. Decio Cortesi, "Un Alchimista del Secolo XVII" (*Nuova Antologia*, 1929, vol. 344), pp. 90, 101.

Chapter 9

1. Tirsi Mario Caffaratto, *La Vita meravigliosa del Cavalier Incognito ossia di Virrorio Cornelio, Comico, Spadaccino, eremita, Ciarlatano e Chirurgo dentista del Re di Sardegna* (Saluzzo: Edizioni Vitalitò, 1966), p. 14.

2. State Archives of Siena, Studio, f. 89, year 1805.

3. Albert Chevalier, "Un charlatan du dix-huitième siècle: Le Grand Thomas" (*Mèmoires de la Societé de l'histoire de Paris, et de l'Ile de France*, 1881), vol. VII, p. 67.

4. Guido Rizzi, "Gli Specifici segreti dei cavadenti del '700 a Venezia" (*Rivista Italiana di Stomatologia*, no. 11, November, 1949), p. 1218.

5. *Ibid.*, p. 1219.

6. *Ibid.*, p. 1221.

7. Alfredo Ilardi, "Processo contro un "Abusivo" esercitante in Roma alla fine del XVII secolo" (*Pagine di Storia della Medicina*, no. 3, May–June, 1965), pp. 69–79.

8. Rizzi, *Gli Specifici segreti dei cavadenti*, op. cit., p. 1226.

9. Vittorio Cavenago, *Di un onorato cavadenti e avventuriero italiano del primo Settecento* (Venice: Zanetti, ed., 1923), p. 16ff.

10. *Ibid.*, p. 18.

11. Colombani Giuseppe da Parma, detto l'Alfier Lombardo, *Il tutto ristretto in poco o sia il tesoro aperto dove ognuno può arrichirsi di virtù, salute e ricchezza* (Venice: Milocco, 1724), p. 29.

12. *Ibid.*, p. 65–67.

13. Tirsi Caffaratto, *La Vita Meravigliosa del Cavalier Incognito ossia di Vittorio Cornelio*, op. cit., p. 35.

14. *Ibid.*, pp. 40–41.

15. *Ibid.*, pp. 44–45.

16. *Ibid.*, pp. 89–90.

17. *Memorie di Carlo Goldoni* (Milan: Edoardo Sonzogno ed., 1876), chap. XXIX, p. 82.

18. Alessandro d'Ancona, *Viaggiatori e Avventurieri* (Florence: Sansoni, 1974), p. 113.

19. Bonafede Vitali, *Lettera scritta ad un Cavaliere suo Padrone dall'Anonimo in difesa della professione del Salimbanco* (Verona: Fratelli Merli, 1732), p. 2ff.

20. *Memorie degli Scrittori e Letterati Parmigiani*, edited by Ireneo Affò and Angelo Pezzana (Bologna: A. Forni, 1883), pp. 107–111.

21. *Memorie di Carlo Goldoni*, op. cit., chap. XXIX, p. 82.

Chapter 10

1. Pietro Aretino, *Lettere*, edited by S. Ortolani (Turin: Einaudi, 1943), p. 167.

2. Paolo Zacchia, *Questiones medico-legales* (Rome: Facciotti, 1628), p. 85.

3. Ottonelli, *Della Christiana Moderazione del Theatro*, see Chap. 2, note 11, p. 3, 448.

4. Emilio Nesi, *Il Diario della Stamperia di Ripoli* (Florence: Seeber, 1903), p. 80.

5. State Archives of Florence, Reggenza, f. 624, insert no. 13.

6. *Gazzetta Toscana*, 1770, no. 48, p. 71.

7. Chiappelli, *I Primordi della Pubblicità Medica in Italia*, see Chap. 5, note 12, p. 135.

8. *Gazzetta Toscana*, 1780, no. 22, p. 26.

9. *Ibid.*, 1779, no. 18.

10. "Quackery in the Past" (*British Medical Journal*, May 27, 1911), p. 1265.

11. *Gazzetta Toscana*, 1769, no. 41, p. 56.

12. *Ibid.*, 1795, nos. 20–23, p. 67.

13. *Ibid.*, 1771, no. 46.

14. *Ibid.*, 1770, no. 35.

15. *Ibid.*, 1770, no. 4, p. 14.

16. *Ibid.*, 1796, no. 2, p. 43.

17. Mauro Randone and Pierluigi Ponti, "Un metodo di cura del '700, le pillole di mercurio di Agostina Belloste" (*Minerva Medica*, 1966, in Varie (miscellaneous), p. 9.

18. Adalberto Pazzini, "Amenità ... o quasi di chirurgia mediovale" (*Progressi di Terapia*, 1938), no. 12, p. 161.

19. *Gazzetta Toscana*, 1772, no. 43, pp. 170–171.

Chapter 11

1. Giorgio Vasari, *Vite dei più illustri pittori*, (Florence: Lorenzo Torrentino, 1550), p. 342.

2. Pomata, *La Promessa di Guarigione*, see Chap. 5, note 8, p. 129.

3. Tissot, *Avviso al Popolo intorno alla Sanità*, see Chap. 5, note 18, p. 216.

4. Mercuri, *Degli errori popolari d'Italia*, see Chap. 1, note 2, p. 269.

5. Ephraim Chambers, *Cyclopedia; or an Universal Dictionary of Arts and Sciences* (London: James and John Knapton, 1738), p. 147.

6. Jean Astruc, *Traité des Maldies vénériennes* (Paris: Guillam Cavelier, 1740), book II, chap. II, pp. 308–312.

7. "L'Orizzonte di Lodovico Antonio Muratori" (*Il Giardino d'Esculapio*, 1950), no. 1, p. 67.

8. Eric Jameson and E. Trimmer, *The Natural History of Quackery* (London: M. Joseph, 1971), pp. 134–135.

9. Garzoni, *La Piazza Universale di tutte le professioni del Mondo*, see Chap. 1, note 8, p. 182.

10. John Rathbone Oliver, "Spontaneous Combustion — A Literary Curiosity" (*Bulletin of the History of Medicine*,1936), no. IV, 7, pp. 559–572.

11. Johann Heinrich Kopp, *Selbstverbrennungen des menschilichen* (Frankfurt: Korpers C. Hermann, 1811), pp. 4–6.

12. *L'Autopiria: storia di un mito*, excerpts from a conference on the study of the history of forensic medicine in Reggio Emilia, May 21, 1983, edited by C.D. Fonseca (Reggio Emilia, Congedo Editore, 1987), p. 132.

13. Rathbone, *Spontaneous Combustion*, op. cit., p. 570.

14. *Sul preteso vero uomo anticombustibile: Osservazioni Fisiche dell'Abate Giorgio Follini Professore di Filosofia e di Fisica e Geometria* (Turin: B. Barberis, 1808), p. 2ff.

15. Loren Pankratz, "Fire Walking and the Persistence of Charlatans" (*Perspects. Biol. Med.*, 1988), no. 31, pp. 291–298.

Chapter 12

1. Mackay, *Memoirs of Extraordinary Popular Delusions*, see Chap. 4, note 3, pp. 307–308.

2. *Ibid.*, pp. 324–325.

3. Thomas Elton, *Fascination or the Art of Electro-Biology, Mesmerism and Clairvoyance* (London: Job Caudwell, 1865), p. 151.

4. Renato Bettica-Giovannini, *Giuseppe Berruti e i Ciarlatani della Medicina* (Turin: "Annali dell'Ospedale Maria Vittoria di Torino," 1976), vol. 19, pp. 235–272.

5. Ada Lonni, "Medici, Ciarlatani e magistrati nell'Italia liberale," in *Storia d'Italia* (Turin: Einuadi, Annali, vol. VII, "Malattia e Medicina," 1984), pp. 822–823.

6. Franco Voltaggio, *L'Arte della guarigione nelle culture umane* (Turin: Bollati e Boringhieri, 1992), pp. 662–663.

7. Bettica-Giovannini, *Giuseppe Berruti e i Ciarlatani della Medicina*, op. cit., p. 246.

8. Corsini, *Medici Ciarlatani e Ciarlatani Medici*, see Chap. 2, note 9, p. 78.

9. Giovan Battista Ughelli, *Medici e Clienti* (Palermo: Ed. Prif., 1911), p. 32.

10. Corsini, *Medici Ciarlatani e Ciarlatani Medici*, see Chap. 2, note 9, pp. 96–97.

11. Arturo Frizzi, *Il Ciarlatano* (Mantova: Tipografia Coop. La Provinciale, 1912), pp. 102–105.

12. *Cambridge Illustrated History of Medicine*, edited by Roy Porter (Cambridge: Cambridge University Press, 1996), p. 62.

13. Ardengo Soffici, *Passi tra le rovine* (Florence: Vallecchi, 1952), p. 117.

14. *Domenica del Corriere*, February, 1912, no. 7, cover page.

15. *Ibid.*, January, 1914, no. 2, p. 6.

16. H. Burger, "The Doctor, the Quack, and the Appetite of the Public for Magic in Medicine," in *Procedures of the Royal Society of Medicine*, November 1, 1933, p. 173.

17. "Il Giardino d'Esculapio," 1950, no. 1, pp. 35–36.

18. *Gazzetta Toscana delle Scienze Medico-Fisiche*, 1845, no. 10, pp. 289–295.

Chapter 13

1. Boccone, *Museo di Fisica e di Esperienze,* see Chap. 4, note 2, pp. 74–75.
2. Fioravanti, *Dello Specchio di Scienza Universale* , see Chap. 6, note 5, p. 283.
3. Mercuri, *Degli errori popolari d'Italia,* see Chap. 1, note 2, p. 310.
4. Mackay, *Memoirs of Extraordinary Popular Delusions,* see Chap. 4, note 3, p. 153.
5. Fioravanti, *De'Capricci Medicinali,* see Chap. 6, note 5, p. 126.
6. Pietro Capparoni, "L'Erbolato: Discorso Reclame per un Medico Ciarlatano fatto da Ludovico Ariosto," Extract from the *Bollettino Storico Italiano dell'Arte Sanitaria,* issue 4, July-August, 1926, p. 18.
7. Sebastiano Benelli, *Il Terror della morte, o sia l'estratto di tutta la medicina curativa* (Venice: Domenico Valvasense, 1707), p. 45.
8. Horacio Jinich, "La verdad y el error en medicina," *Gazeta Medica de Mexico,* 1984, 120, no. 4, pp. 138–141.
9. Jean Paul Escandre, *Mirages de la Médicine* (Paris: Albin Michel, 1987), pp. 71–72.
10. Serge Voronoff, *A Study of the Means of Restoring Vital Energy* (Sydney: Allen G. & Udvin Ltd., 1923), p. 16.
12. Fioravanti, *Della Fisica,* see Chap. 6, note 1, p. 338.

Chapter 14

1. Quoted by E. Reza, *Note a Scipione Mercurii* (Padova: Tipografia G.B. Raudi, 1902), p. 16.
2. Mercuri, see Chap. 1, note 2, p. 270.
3. Cosimo Aldana, *Discorso contro il Volgo* (Florence: Giorgio Marescotti, 1578), p. 231.
4. Matteo Bandello, *Le Novelle,* edited by G. Brognoligo (Bari: Laterza, 1910).
5. Erasmus of Rotterdam, quoted in *Il Giardino di Esculapio,* no. 4, October, 1936, XIV, p. 34.
6. Benedicenti, *Malati, Medici e Farmacisti,* see Chap. 4, note 1, p. 1035.
7. Gandini, *Avviso al Popolo,* see Chap. 5, note 18, p. 213.
8. Jean Baptiste Poquelin, alias Molière, *Le Malade Imaginaire* (Paris: Booking Int., 1993), Troisième Intermédie, Act III, Sc. XIV, p. 243.
9. Giov. Maria Bonardo Fratteggiano, *Della Miseria et Eccellenza della Vita Umana: Ragionamenti due* (Venice: Fabio e Agostino Zoppini, 1536), pp. 109–110.
10. Isabelle Stengers, *Medici e Stregoni,* Italian translation byAlfredo Salsano (Turin: Bollati Boringheri, 1995), p. 124.
11. Joseph Fursay-Fusswerk, "La Chute des Idoles" in *Sciences de l'homme* (Toulouse: private ed., 1986), p. 121.

Index

243